Contents

Preface

Observation of vocal fold vibration should be a standard part of the clinical repertoire of speech pathologists and laryngologists interested in voice production. Visual perceptual judgments need not be threatening to clinicians! Underlying all clinical judgments of vocal fold vibration are a few basic concepts of the anatomical structure and mechanical properties. If these concepts are thoroughly understood, the different vibratory characteristics can be appreciated as diagnostic and prognostic signs of vocal health.

Our intent in writing this text is to gradually and logically develop a comprehensive view of what constitutes vocal fold vibration, to ensure that all clinicians be able to make meaningful interpretations of vibratory characteristics, and to relate these interpretations to videostroboscopic observations of the larynx.

The content and illustrative examples of this text reflect the authors' view that stroboscopic examination of vocal fold vibration helps provide a unified concept of structure and function. The laryngeal system must be fully understood in its static anatomical sense and in its kinetic function before abnormalities can be recognized. Knowledge of structure and function are prerequisite to understanding the significance of the abnormal changes in function — as seen with videostroboscopy — that go hand-in-hand with structural lesions and other etiologies of dysphonia. Similarly, the tools used for examining the structure and function must be understood to achieve the best results and to avoid errors in interpreting video recordings.

Thus, this book provides a short and basic but comprehensive survey of the structure of the larynx and of the development and application of the videostroboscope. The chapters lead the clinician from a basic description of the histological and mechanical properties of the larynx to the more complicated interpretations of the relation between movement and other clinical findings. Moreover, the planning and arrangement of the chapters guide the clinician reading the entire text in learning how to make informed decisions on selection of equipment and development of a clinical protocol that will meet his or her needs. Readers are referred to manufacturers and current literature for specific information on methods of selection and combination of equipment. Technology changes too rapidly to include such information in a basic text.

Information on videostroboscopy in this clinical text is presented through numerous illustrations and discussed in a didactic, positive manner principally from the authors' viewpoints. Some parts of the text are intentionally redundant. We are of the belief that redundancy facilitates learning. The number of individual citations is small and selective, but the text is based on voluminous literature, as indicated in the Bibliography, as well as on personal experience.

We hope that clinicians will find this book useful in their practice with individuals with voice disorders.

Acknowledgments

Writing a book involves many people in addition to the authors; few can write a book alone. We wish to acknowledge our considerable debt to our colleagues, editors, students, secretaries, patients, and teachers. To them we owe incalculable debt for their teachings and for their inspiration in the conception and development of this clinical text. It is our pleasure to recognize the specific contributions of individuals who helped in the preparation of this book: our secretaries Yasuko Takahashi, Deb Milbauer, and Kate Emerick, who helped type the manuscript; our editor Celeste Kirk who helped improve the manuscript and make it more readable; our illustrator, Joan Kozel, who helped Diane M. Bless with some of the illustrations; and our students Kate Bunton and Molly Strittmater, who helped track down obscure references and meet Federal Express deadlines. Additionally, several individuals have given us permission to refer to their work in detail in this book, including Drs. R. E. (Ed) Stone, Jr., Janina Casper, Raymond Colton, Peak Woo, David Brewer, and H. P. Olson. Their words added depth to this book and made it a more valuable clinical reference. Finally, we would be remiss without making special mention of Marie Linvill, the Singular in-house editor for her patience and persistent belief that the book would be completed.

CHAPTER

1

Introduction and Historical Review

Abnormal vocal fold vibration both contributes to the development of laryngeal pathology and results from the presence of pathology (Childers, 1977; Hirano, 1981b; von Leden, Moore, & Timcke, 1960b). Vocal dysfunction can be evaluated by techniques relying on perceptual, aerodynamic, or acoustic measures. However, the abnormal vocal fold vibration that contributes to dysphonia can remain undetected by those indirect measurement techniques (Ludlow, 1981). This might be true, at least in part, because, for most evaluative techniques, clinicians must infer what given vibratory characteristics are on the basis of their observations of the speech waveform. A notable exception is videostroboscopy, whereby a permanent image of the apparent motion of the vocal folds is recorded to evaluate a variety of phonatory conditions.

Videostroboscopy is one of the most practical techniques currently available for clinical examination of the larynx. It is a technique that provides useful information concerning the nature of vibration, an immediate image of the presence or absence of pathology, and a permanent record. When videostroboscopy is used by trained observers in conjunc-

tion with other assessment techniques, it can provide both qualitative and quantitative data on vocal function and dysfunction.

Vocal dysfunction can be caused by impairment of the movement of any part of the larynx. Normal vibration requires that the vocal fold be soft and pliable, that the border be free of irregularities, and that the ligament have adequate laxity to permit motion. Additional requirements include that stiffness be sufficient to maintain natural elastic properties, that the cricoarytenoid joints permit movement in all directions necessary for phonation, and that an adequate steady driving pressure be provided by the respiratory system. Impairment of the folds, ligaments, or joints can result in disruption of normal vibratory relationships.

Most important in understanding dysfunction is a knowledge of normal voice production (see Chapter 2). Accurate evaluation of voice disorders demands knowledge of functional anatomy and of those factors that contribute to normal and abnormal movement patterns. The examiner who does not understand the normal vocal mechanism cannot discern abnormal deviations or understand the mechanism of a disorder. In the absence of an understanding of functional anatomy, the picture tells no story, the examination becomes meaningless, and the recommended treatment might fail. Therefore, this book presents information on vocal fold anatomy and on normal and disordered voice production, as well as on the principles and theory of stroboscopy.

CONCEPT AND DEFINITION OF STROBOSCOPY

The noun stroboscope has come to mean a particular type of optical instrument; the adjective stroboscopic is applied to any pulsating light phenomenon. It refers to the use of intermittent illumination to aid in the process of observation.

The concept of the stroboscope is closely allied with that of high-speed camera photography motion picture. There are good reasons for this: Both have evolved from the same process; both permit observation of movement/motion; and both permit the observer to freeze motion. In high-speed photography, the camera "freezes" motion by a rapid sampling process. This process employs constant light to record images in frames on film, which is developed and subsequently sequentially projected for the observer to interpret. The motion picture projector recreates the original movement by the rapid presentation of successive samples. The stroboscope process is identical, except that intermittent flashes of light "frame" the action and the eye or a video camera can substitute for the film. In that case, interpretation of the results is immediate. Although the two processes differ, both operate on the basis of sampling and both produce optical illusions. High-speed photography has the advantage of capturing more frames of motion per unit time than videostroboscopy. Videostroboscopy has the advantage of being less expensive, providing on-line visualization of motion, allowing for larger protocols, and being easier to use.

A stroboscope, then, can be described as an instrument used to study the phases of motion by means of a light source that is periodically interrupted or pulsed. The intervals between the flashes can be regulated, and multiple exposures of moving objects can be made. Thus, stroboscopy is an optical

phenomenon based on Talbot's Law that captures fragments of complete movement (Figure 1–1). As a result, objects moving rapidly appear to stand still or to move only slowly. To understand how these fragments of complete movement yield an apparent image of the total event, it is necessary to consider the limitations in human vision, along with the function of light and illusion of movement.

Talbot's Law

When the human eye is presented with an image, the image lingers on the retina for 0.2 seconds after exposure. This is called *persistence of vision.*

Because the eye can perceive no more than five distinct images per second, sequential images produced at intervals shorter than 0.2 seconds persist on the retina and fuse with successive images to produce the optical illusion of *apparent motion.* This phenomenon, called Talbot's Law, explains how we see a series of rapidly changing still images on a motion picture film strip as one continuous moving picture (cited in Harley, 1988).

Furthermore, when the motion of an intermittently seen object is ambiguous, the visual system resolves confusion by applying tricks that reflect an individual's built-in knowledge of properties of the physical world. In other words, when the visual system is confronted with a rapid series of still images, the mind can "fill in" the gaps between "frames" and imagine that it sees an object in continuous motion.

To perceive an intermittently visible object (e.g., the beating of a bird's wings), the visual system must detect what is called *correspondence.* That is, it must determine which parts of successive images reflect a single object in motion. If each picture differs only slightly from the one before it, the visual system can perceive motion; if successive pictures differ noticeably, the motion appears jerky, as in early cinematography. Therefore, if successive images differing only slightly from each other are presented more rapidly than every 0.2 second, the viewer will use his or her innate, unconscious knowledge of the world to fill in the gaps and perceive apparent motion of an object.

A natural corollary of these observations is that a clear image of an object vibrating too rapidly to be visible to the naked eye could be captured by illumi-

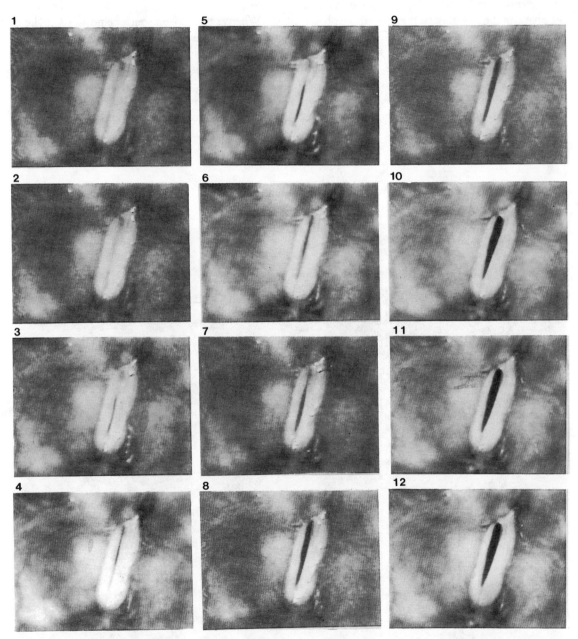

Figure 1-1. Sampling fragments of vibration. Reading the frames in sequence, one can easily visualize the closed glottis in frame 1, beginning to open in frame 4, opening by frame 8, closing slightly in frame 9, and maximally open in frame 12.

nating the object with intermittent short flashes of light (Figure 1–2). Flashes of light in synchrony with the phases of the vibratory cycle expose those phases at a rate visible by the naked eye. Thus, by missing part of a rapid event and filling in with our visual persistence, we are able to see the movements of bird's wings, or the moment of a rip of paper occurring at the penetration site of an arrow in a target, and other such events occurring too rapidly to visually process with normal lighting.

Light and Illusion of Movement

Whereas typical light sources emit an AC pulse of light or DC continuous light (Figure 1–3A), the stroboscopic light emits rapid pulses (Figure 1–3B), each pulse illuminates a point of the vibratory cycle. Illuminated points are visually fused, providing an averaged vibratory pattern over successive cycles (Figure 1–4).

Light pulses can be emitted at the same frequency as the vibration or at a slight variation in frequency.

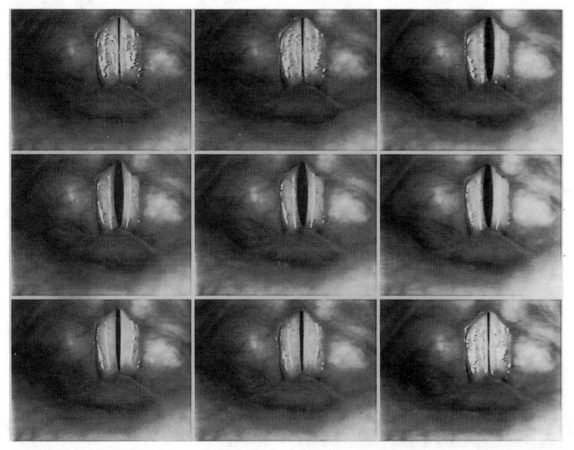

Figure 1–2. Videostroboscopic print of one cycle of vibration. Opening of the glottis differs slightly from frame to frame. If the images were presented in rapid succession rather than in its current flat form, the observer would perceive motion and fill in the visual gaps.

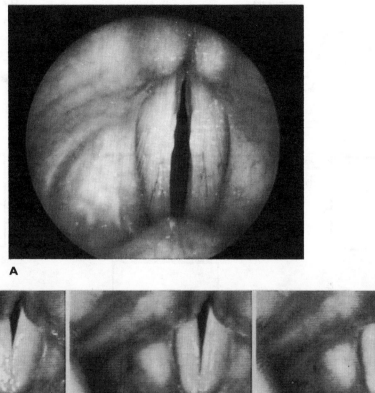

A

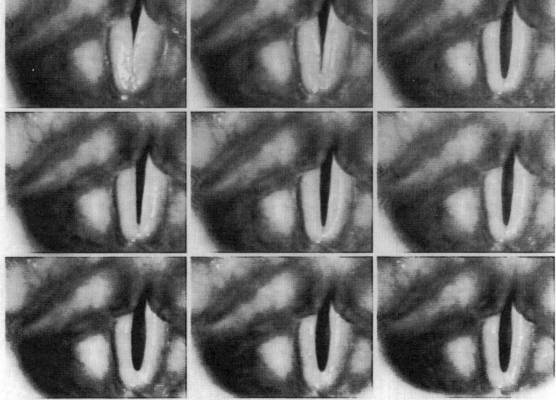

B

Figure 1-3. Images captured by a constant light source (A) are different than those captured by videostroboscopic light source (B).

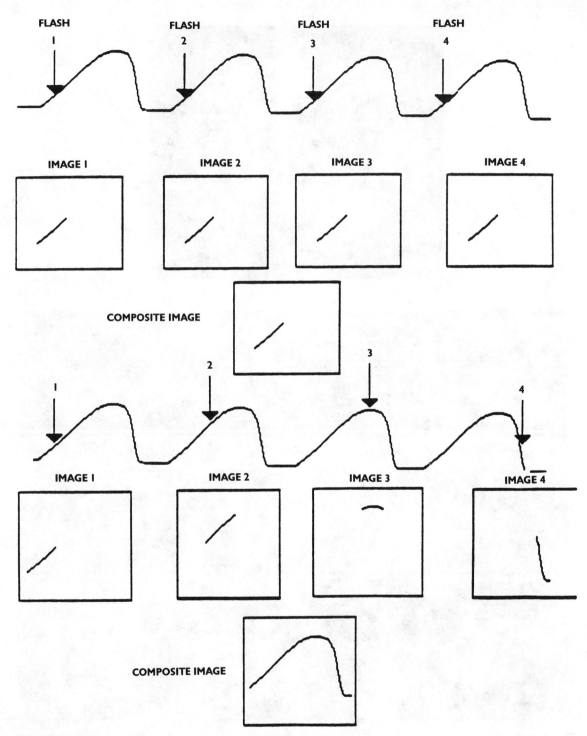

Figure 1-4. Parts of the vibratory curve are sampled to produce a fused image of motion under observation. In the upper part of the figure, the light pulses are regular and produced at the same frequency of vibration, motion appears to stand still. In the lower part, the pulses are regular but differ 1.5 Hz from the frequency of vibration. A motion is observed.

Synchronization — production of identical frequency — of illumination with the frequency of vibration results in apparent freezing of motion (Figure 1–5). A frozen image allows scrutiny of an object (in laryngoscopy, of course, the vocal folds) in any position of the cycle. In such a frozen state, any appearance of movement indicates that the vibration of the object is aperiodic (Figure 1–6) or asymmetrical (Figure 1–7). Varying the frequency of illumination by 1 to 2 hertz (Hz) from that of the vibration (Figure 1–8) causes each successive light impulse to strike successive phases of the vibratory cycle. This systematic phase shift along the cycles results in a slow-motion effect as recorded on video frames.

The sequential frames provide a visual image of one cycle — an optical illusion of apparent motion. Thus, one cycle of vibration captured on standard video frames is actually obtained from several cycles of vibration (Figure 1–9). Standard video recorders record at 33 frames/second, which means a typical male recording at 100 Hz would record a fragment of vibration approximately every four cycles. Thus, illusion of movement offers the best mode to date for studying vibratory movement.

HISTORY OF STROBOSCOPY

Development of Stroboscopy

Historically, stroboscopy is not new. Harley (1988) and Kivenson (1965) have written marvelous and illuminating histories of the optical events that relate to the development of modern stroboscopy; a combined synopsis appears here. Optical illusions have fascinated humans for eons. Prehistoric cultures were probably alarmed by the illusion of motion of stationary objects caused by flickering camp fires. In all likelihood, curiosity eventually replaced fear, and people developed a desire to create this kind of optical illusion. The earliest attempts to control and use optical phenomena were probably

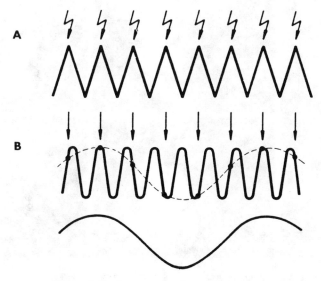

Figure 1–5. A train of pulses: (A) Synchronized flash intervals result in the point of illumination occurring at the same point of each cycle and an apparently motionless image; and (B) When flash intervals occur at a slightly faster rate, illumination progresses along each pulse and results in apparent slow motion.

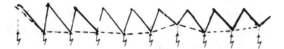

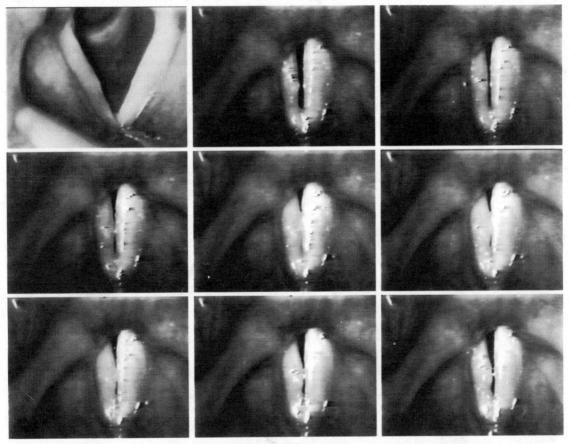

Figure I-6. Aperiodic vibration can result in apparent motion when the image should be frozen. The vibration is generally irregular, jerky, and of small magnitude.

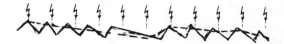

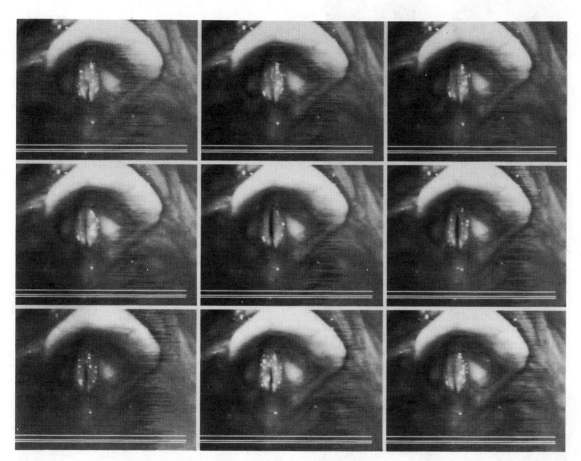

Figure 1–7. Asymmetrical vibration can result in apparent motion when the image should be frozen. The amplitude of lateral movement is small. The movement may be flutter-like in appearance.

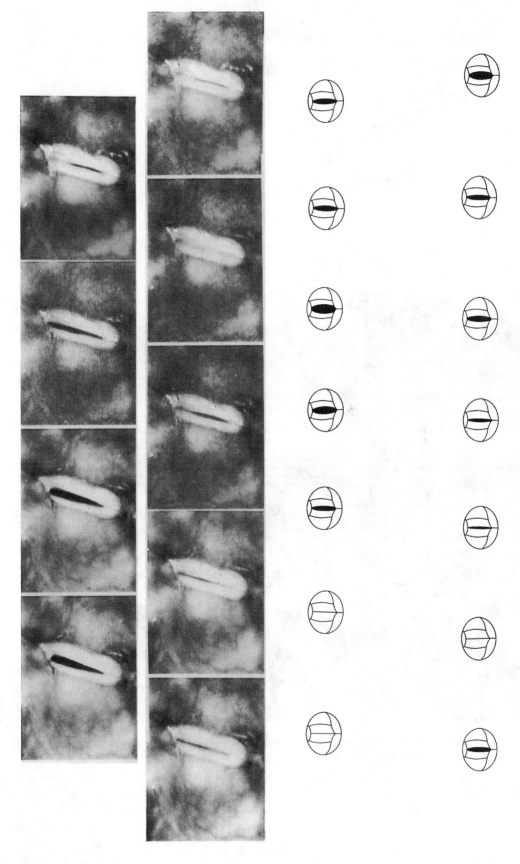

Figure 1–8. Stroboscopic illumination can provide a slow-motion effect as would be the case with these illustrations if they were presented in rapid succession as with a flick book. The top of the figure contains video frames and the bottom diagramatic depictions are of the superior view of the larynx. The bottom illustrates how increased frame rate provides more information about the cycle.

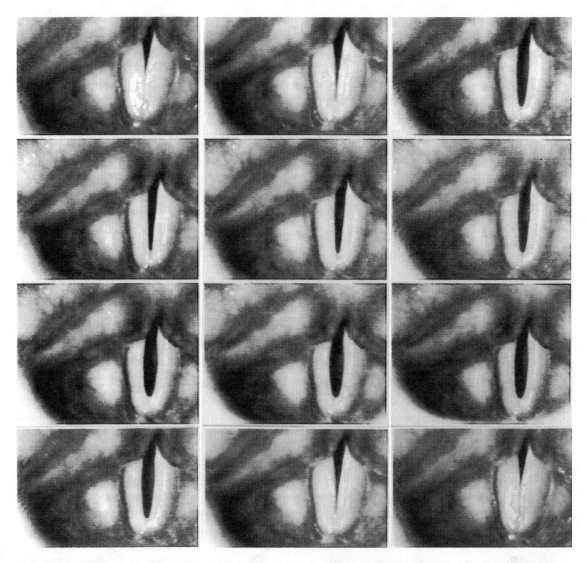

Figure 1-9. One cycle of vibration captured on video frames represents sampling from several cycles of vibration.

linked to magic and religion, possibly stemming from flickering shadows thrown by torchlight or shafts of sunlight deep in caves or tombs. The ancient Greeks are said to have painted a number of successive poses of a dancing figure on the vertical columns of one of their temples and to have galloped at high speed past the pictures. To the horseman, the pictures appeared to be a single person moving continuously and performing a dance.

Some of the groundwork for studying optical phenomena was done as early as the 17th century by Sir Isaac Newton (cited in Harley, 1988, p. 21) who used the phenomenon that would become known as *persistence of vision* to demonstrate the composition of white light. Another demonstration showed that the retina of the eye could tire. If a subject stared at a simple, high-contrast picture for a minute or so in bright light and then looked at a white wall, the "tired" retina would generate a negative impression of the picture. Both of these observations were fundamental to developing the early pictorial representations of movement.

People have long recognized that the appearance of objects changes when they are viewed in mirrors and through lenses. Interest in optics produced telescopes, microscopes, and magic lanterns by the 18th century, but no significant investigation of apparent motion effects occurred until the 19th century. The Industrial Revolution, newly-acquired leisure, and popular interest in scientific novelties led to the scientific study of many optical illusions, including those of moving objects.

Two investigations in England in the early 19th century were critical to the development of the stroboscope. In 1825, Roget, father of the thesaurus, published a paper (Kivenson, 1965) describing the appearance of rotating carriage spokes when viewed through a picket fence: The wheel seemed to move horizontally without rotation, and the spokes appeared curved but stationary.

Talbot's Law of "persistence of vision" and the concept of "correspondence" led to the development of a host of popular and ingenious moving picture/optical toys, as well as of scientific instruments. It is not clear whether the toys fostered development of the instruments or vice versa, but it is clear that the principles of development were the same and the times were roughly parallel.

The first optical motion toy to make use of the two principles was the thaumatrope (from the Greek "thaumato," meaning marvel or wonder and "trope," meaning circle), invented by Dr. J.A. Paris in 1827 (Harley, 1988). It was a small square card with a string attached to both sides and a series of drawings on each side, depicting, for example, a clown turning a somersault. When the card was spun in a circle by twisted cords, the series produced the optical illusion of continuous action (Figure 1–10).

In Belgium, Joseph Plateau (1830) developed a compact form of the Greek "motion picture," which he dubbed the phenakistoscope (Harley, 1988). Images representing successive stages of motion were drawn around the periphery of a rotatable disk (Figure 1–11) and separated by slits. The instrument was held up to a mirror, set spinning, and the figures were observed in the mirror by sighting through the moving slits. The shutter-like effect of the passage of slits provided the flashes of light that illuminated the images. Later, Plateau developed disks that produced illusions of contraction or expansion depending on which direction they were rotated (Figure 1–11).

In 1831, Faraday produced an "illusion of arrested motion" instrument (Kivenson, 1965) (Figure 1–12). Two slotted cardboard disks were mounted on friction drives to permit rotation in opposite directions. A black background was placed behind the disk furthest from the viewer. The line of sight of the observer was such that one disk was viewed through the other disk by sighting in a line parallel to the rotational axis. When the disks were rotated fast enough, the individual spokes appeared blurred and the original number of spokes was doubled, with the motion appearing to be arrested. This optical illusion was explained by Helmholtz (1948) as the result of the difference in illumination over only two intensity levels: When the spokes are aligned (a front spoke blocking a rear spoke), the black background can be seen and overall illumination is at a minimum. When the disk positions are staggered, the observer sees two sets of relatively bright spokes and no background. The latter condition results in the greatest illumination and the image is visually retained on the retina to produce the illusion of stopped motion.

At about the same time, Stampfer, a Viennese scientist, independently developed disks for observing apparent motion (Kivenson, 1965). He called his instrument a stroboscope and that word is still used to connote any pulsating light generated to observe motion.

The devices developed by Faraday, Plateau, and Stampfer are, physiologically, true stroboscopes because they make use of the same response mechanism in the observer, although the outcomes are opposite.

Also, at about the same time, the zoetrope ("zoe" is Greek for life) was invented in England by William Horner (cited in Kivenson, 1965) (Figure 1–13); it was rediscovered and patented by Milton Bradley in the United States in 1867. This device consisted of a spinning drum inside a spinning cylinder. A series of pictures on interchangeable strips of paper could be slipped inside the drum. The illusion of movement was created when the series of drawings was viewed

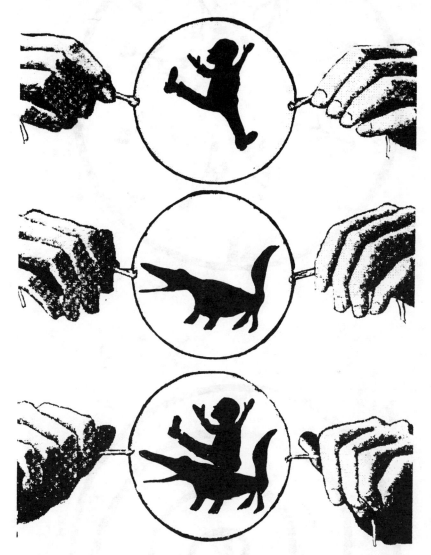

Figure 1–10 "Thaumatrope" was one of the first known optical toys to capitalize on persistence of vision. A cardboard disk with pictures on each side has short strings tied to the edge. When twirled, the picture on one side appears to be superimposed on the other, so that in the thaumatrope illustrated the man rides the alligator. Thus, when the disk is twirled rapidly, instead of seeing an alligator and a man separately, we see the man sitting on the back of the alligator, as shown in the bottom picture in the drawing. In other words, as we twirl the disk the image of the alligator is thrown on the retina, and before it can disappear the man is thrown on the same retina screen, and so the man and alligator appear together, giving the continuous illusion of a man riding an alligator. This toy may have been the scientific inspiration for moving pictures.

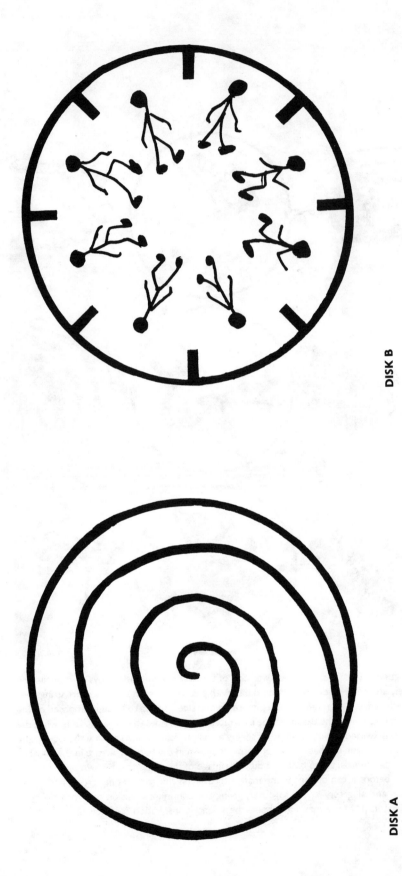

DISK A

DISK B

Figure I–II. Two types of disks referred to as the "phenakistoscope," developed by Plateau for "motion pictures." When spun, the lines on the disk in A appear to move toward the periphery of the disk. In B, the evolution of the phenakistoscope to the "fantascope" is illustrated. Use of mirrors and slits around the periphery for viewing the images resulted in moving pictures.

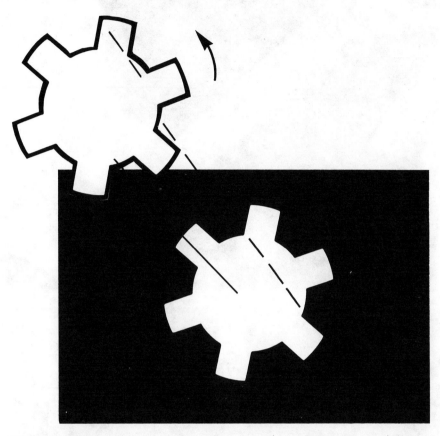

Figure 1–12. In 1831, Faraday developed an instrument (shown here in schematic) for producing "illusion of arrested motion." Two slotted cardboard disks were mounted to permit rotation in opposite directions. A black background was placed behind the disk furthest from the observer. When the disks were spun sufficiently fast, individual spokes appeared blurred. By viewing the spokes parallel to the rotational axes, the observer would see a stationary wheel. The spokes appeared blurred with double the number of either wheel, and motion appeared to be arrested.

through slits as the viewer set the cylinder spinning. A "build-your-own" zoetrope is found in the Appendix near the back of this book (Groenenings, 1991).

In these toys, the viewer caught a brief glimpse of each picture, but because the disk or drum was in continuous motion, the definition was poor; and as the glimpse was brief, the pictures were dark. A number of improvements were tried with varying success. By the mid-19th century, scientists wrote about the design considerations affecting strobe ob-

servations. The various relations between available light, motion blur, field of view, and pulse duration continued to be factors in the development of modern strobes and associated hardware accessories.

The first major advance occurred in 1877 when Emile Reynauds used mirrors in what he called a prakinoscope (the Greek "praxis" means action) (Harley, 1988). He used a drum of rectangular mirrors, one per picture, to reflect the zoetrope picture strips. The diameter of the mirror drum was half that of the picture drum and thus the reflected images

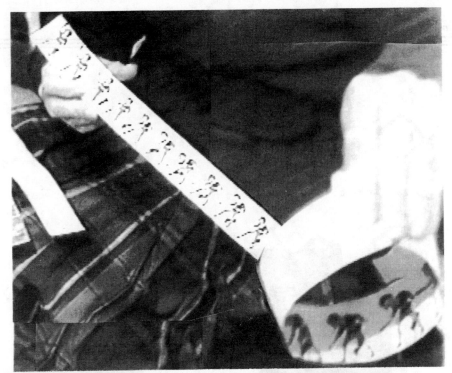

A

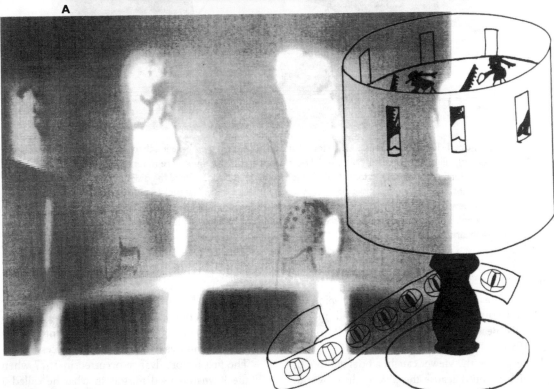

B

Figure 1-13. Horner's "zoetrope" introduced more moving parts that led to technical advances in the use of light for viewing images. The cylinder with pictures mount- ed on strips placed inside, rotated on a pivot, and the ob- server viewing through slits as they came quickly before his or her eyes, saw the figures in action.

appeared to be at the center. Whereas the zoetrope had allowed only about 10% of the light to pass through the slits, the prakinoscope mirrors reflected about 90%, providing a clearer, brighter picture.

By 1900, many German toymakers offered zoetropes and prakinoscopes operated either by tiny electric motors or by steam engines, and "flick" books whose pages of successive images were riffled by the thumb to create apparent motion (Harley, 1988). Whereas their major function was entertainment, these also were important laboratory instruments. Some of these devices are thought to have led to the invention of the cinema in the 1890s, and to early experiments with television in the 1920s and 1930s. Without the technological advances in television recording devices, the stroboscope would not be the clinical tool it is today.

Scientific Applications

The original stroboscopes devolved from the of Roget, Faraday, Plateau, and Stampfer were mechanical and somewhat cumbersome and did not work well under poor ambient light conditions.

As early as 1836, Plateau had suggested the use of an intermittent spark (driven by a tuning fork contractor) to illuminate moving objects and to obtain stationary patterns for study (Harley, 1988). Nearly 100 years after these suggestions, H. E. Edgerton and his associates (Edgerton, 1970) developed gas discharge tubes for stroboscopy from which evolved many of the principles of modern stroboscopic instrumentation. The Edgerton group was also the first to use an oscillator to control the frequency of discharge and the flashing rate.

Initially the stroboscopic method was used in physics for the study of periodic oscillations of bodies to demonstrate vibrations of strings and reeds and for observation of other objects with high frequencies of motion. The notion that the stroboscopic method could be used in medicine was first conceived by Doppler (cited in Oertel, 1895). The early medical stroboscopes were mechanical: A disk perforated on the periphery was used in conjunction with a clockwork motor. The motor rotated the disk at right angle to a light beam as the light was directed

onto a moving object. When a perforation passed in front of the light, the effect was a pulsed light.

The use of a stroboscopic light source for examining the larynx has almost as long a history as that of the continuous light source reportedly first used by Manuel Garcia (1855). Only 24 years later, Oertel (1895), an internist, used a stroboscopic light source with a laryngeal mirror (laryngostroboscopy) for investigating voice production in different registers. Oertel's mechanical system used a hand-cranked, perforated, rotating disk to interrupt the beam of light.

Two types of stroboscopic lights, then, were used for scientific purposes: The first was mechanical (Figure 1–14), using a constant light with the period of observation controlled by a shutter placed between the source of light and the object being observed, and the other used a special intermittent gas light that was capable of producing instantaneous flashes, at exposures of millionths of a second. The period of observation was controlled by the duration of the light flashes.

Application of the stroboscopy to the vibrating vocal folds resulted in the movements appearing to be arrested or to be in slow motion. With the stroboscope, the examiner was able to use the "frozen" position of the vocal folds, at will, by synchronizing the light pulses with the frequency of vibration. The examiner could make detailed observations of the structure in the open or closed position. The illusion of slowmotion was achieved when the rate of illumination was varied slightly in relation to the frequency of vibration, such that each successive light impulse struck a different phase of the vibratory cycle.

Historically, this intermittent effect was achieved in a number of ways: at the source of illumination, between the illumination and the eye, at the eye, and between the eye and the vibrating vocal folds. Whatever the means, the ability to observe motion of the vocal fold was intriguing and stimulated numerous investigations. However, the mechanical (disk) stroboscope was fraught with problems: It was cumbersome and noisy; it could only be used with trained subjects who were able to match the frequency of rotation (and even trained subjects had difficulty maintaining a pitch for the prolonged periods necessary for observation); the frequency of interruption

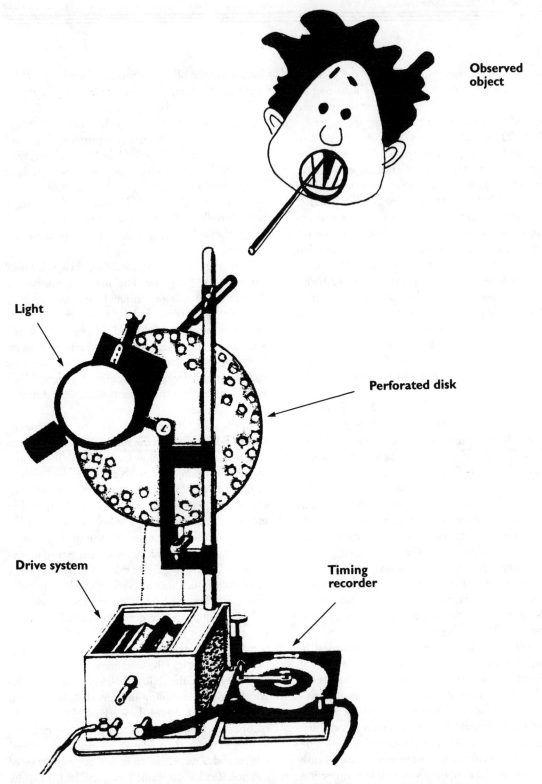

Observed object

Light

Perforated disk

Drive system

Timing recorder

Figure 1–14. Early mechanical stroboscopes used a perforation in front of a constant light source to pulse the light.

was limited to about 1/500 of a second; and the mechanical interruption of light meant considerable loss of illumination and generally poor images. Clinicians would be unsure whether to attribute visible vocal irregularities to the apparatus, patient, or examiner. Consequently, this stroboscope was not embraced by the scientific community. Nevertheless, it was the beginning of an improved means of examining the larynx, particularly for voice production and laryngeal pathologies.

THE MODERN LARYNGOSTROBOSCOPE

Frustrated by the problems associated with the disk type of stroboscopes, many investigators sought to develop a stroboscopic system with a light pulse driven by the patient's own voice. Very quickly, light pulsed at the source became the preferred mode. Early pioneers included Dr. J.W. van den Berg at the University of Groningen, Dr. Rolf Timcke at Hamburg, Dr. Hans von Leden at the University of California at Los Angeles, and Dr. Elimar Schonharl in Erlanger, who wrote the first definitive book (Schonharl, 1960b) on stroboscopic examination of the larynx.

The electronic stroboscopes developed in the 1950s operated on the same principles as the earlier mechanical versions but used a microphone placed on the patient's neck to direct the sound waves. The fundamental frequency of the sound produced in the larynx was transmitted via electronic pulses to a xenon lamp, which emitted a pulsed flash at the same rate; the light flashes corresponded to the frequency of vocal fold vibration. The beam of light was reflected off the head mirror onto the larynx, as in any indirect laryngoscopy. A foot pedal attachment permitted the examiner to make a slight adjustment to the flashes to obtain either a stationary image at any phase of vibration or the typical slow-motion effect.

The advantages of this electronic stroboscope driven by the patient's voice were obvious. Investigators and clinicians were able to see the larynx in motion and to learn about the complex role played by the mucous membrane of the vocal folds, closure patterns, and the impact of various laryngeal pathologies. Use of the stroboscopic equipment quickly became standard practice in European and Japanese clinics, but not in America. Failure to include stroboscopic examinations in routine evaluations of the larynx in the United States no doubt resulted from a number of factors, the least of which was that technological advances were slow, the available equipment was expensive and bulky, there were no standards for observation, and no permanent recording could be made.

In 1977, Yoshida's report on a stroboscopic videotape recording system ushered in worldwide acceptance of the stroboscope as a vital clinical tool for those interested in voice production. The system produced high-quality permanent images that could be viewed by an audience, reviewed with the patient, used for teaching, and used to compare recordings made at different points in time to help determine the progress of treatment. Although the system was expensive, it heralded a new era in stroboscopy. The images were recorded on a standard recorder at 33 frames per second, which meant the image was a composite averaged over several cycles to provide the viewer with an optical illusion of one cycle of vibration. This composite image presented no problems in reviewing normal speakers, but created new challenges for the validity of recordings made on speakers with severe perturbation.

Expense and image quality have changed as a function of mass market demand for high-quality, home video machines and technological developments in optics. New, small, low-light-level, inexpensive, home video cameras have made quality permanent recordings affordable for most clinicians. Other technical advances have made the equipment easy to use (even for the novice) and have made it possible to study the larynx during a variety of phonatory conditions, making stroboscopy truly practical as a routine clinical examination. Ease of use and affordability of equipment have resulted in a large body of literature increasing our knowledge of the physiology of the vocal folds in health and disease. The permanent recordings have also made it possible to train clinicians to use standard procedures for data recording and analysis, which, in turn, permits both intra- and interclinic comparisons.

Most recently, investigators at the Institute of Logopedics and Phoniatrics in Tokyo, led by Dr. Hajime Hirose have developed a high-speed computerized video recording system (Hirose, 1988). The system allows one to observe each cycle of vibration, thereby providing information on irregular cycle-to-cycle variations. The trade-off for obtaining information on each cycle of vibration is some loss in detail and quality of theimage. This is likely to change in the future with advances in resolution of recorders, cameras, and computer systems, and this technique holds much promise for future examination of the larynx.

With these developments, stroboscopy has become a routine part of the examination of individuals with voice disorders in many parts of the world.

Nevertheless, in the final analysis, the capabilities of videostroboscopy rely on the skill of clinicians and their knowledge of voice production. Proper evaluation of disorders demands a comprehensive understanding of vocal fold vibration.

STUDY QUESTIONS

1. What advantages does videostroboscopic examination of the laryrnx provide over other assessment techniques for evaluation of vocal fold vibration?

   a. Videostroboscopy provides more detail regarding cycle-to-cycle variations.

   b. Videostroboscopy provides a direct image of the larynx, making it less likely one has to infer what causes abnormal vibation.

   c. Videostroboscopy provides more repeatable results.

   d. Videostroboscopy is more quantitative than other techniques.

2. What are the vocal fold requirements for normal vocal fold vibration? (Choose as many as apply.)

   a. Soft vocal fold tissue.

   b. Pliable vocal fold tissue.

   c. Glottal margin smooth.

   d. Ligament permits motion.

   e. Glottal margin convex in shape.

3. Videostroboscopy and high-speed photography of the larynx: (Choose as many as apply)

   a. Obtain identical images

   b. Differ in the number of frames per cycle obtained.

   c. Both provide images of laryngeal vibration.

   d. Both provide detail of cycle-to-cycle variation.

   e. Come from the Greek words meaning "to rotate" and "target."

4. Persistence of vision refers to

   a Any method that makes a permanent recording of a visual input.

   b. Lingering of a visual image on the retina.

   c. Filling in the gaps visual frames.

   d. Our ability to perceive intermittently visible objects.

   e. Apparent motion.

5. How does stroboscopic light differ from standard light sources?

   a. Stroboscopic light source is DC continuous light.

   b. Stroboscopic light source is brighter.

   c. Stroboscopic light source is pulsating.

   d. Stroboscopic light source is AC.

   e. Stroboscopic light source is incandescent.

6. Synchronization refers to:

   a. Production of pulses of light varying the frequency of illumination by 1 to 2 hertz from that of vibration.

b. Production of pulses of illumination at the same rate as vibration.

c. Matching the frequency of illumination to an outside stimulus.

d. Matching the frequency of illumination and vocal fold vibration in such a way that apparent motion is recorded.

e. Timing characteristics of the internal clock in the stroboscope.

7. Toys have had historical significance in the development of stroboscopy because:

a. They used the same principles and led to development of modern stroboscopy.

b. They provided leisure time to the scientists to help clear their minds for other developments.

c. They provided the funds necessary to develop the scientific instruments.

d. They demonstrated that even little children could make use of apparent motion.

e. They helped illuminate the phenomenon of optical illusion.

8. The original stroboscopes were:

a. Mechanical and cumbersome.

b. Connected to high-speed photography.

c. Driven by the patient's voice.

d. Used most frequently in the United States.

e. Essentially identical to those used today.

9. The advantages of electronic stroboscopes are:

a. The stroboscope can be driven by the voice.

b. The system isn't as fast and therefore can make better use of the persistence of vision.

c. Few.

d. Not immediately obvious.

2

Vocal Fold Vibration

STRUCTURE OF THE VOCAL FOLD

Knowledge of vocal fold vibration is essential to successful examination of the larynx by videostroboscopy. Recognizing vibratory patterns exhibited by vocal folds in general leads the clinician to the appreciation of individual characteristics of vocal folds in action. Familiarity with normal patterns provides the basis for recognizing and identifying the characteristics of the abnormal voice and for diagnosing and treating it properly. Assessing the vibratory behavior of the vocal fold begins with a thorough understanding of the vocal fold structure.

STRUCTURE OF THE VOCAL FOLD

Knowledge of the structural composition of the vocal folds is the key not only to comprehending the vibratory behavior, but also appreciating how deviations in the normal structure resulting from pathologies cause changes in the vibratory characteristics.

In the human adult vocal fold (Figure 2–1), the area at and around the edge of the vocal fold moves most markedly during phonation. Likewise, it is in this area that a vocal fold lesion will make the greatest perceptual difference in voice production. From a histological point of view, this area consists of five layers:

1. The epithelium of the mucosa, which is of the squamous cell type. From a mechanical point of view, the epithelium can be regarded as a thin shell with the purpose of maintaining the shape of the vocal fold;

2. The superficial layer of the lamina propria of the mucosa, which primarily consists of loose fibers and matrix. It is referred to as Reinke's space. From a mechanical point of view, this layer is very pliable and can be regarded as somewhat like a mass of soft gelatin;

3. The intermediate layer of the lamina propria of the mucosa, which primarily consists of elastic fibers. The fibers run approximately parallel to the edge of the vocal fold. From a mechanical point of view, this layer can be likened to a bundle of soft rubber bands;

4. The deep layer of the lamina propria of the mucosa, which consists chiefly of collagenous fibers. The fibers run almost parallel to the edge of the vocal fold. From a mechanical point of view, this layer is akin to a bundle of cotton threads; and

5. The vocalis muscle, which constitutes the main body of the vocal fold. The muscle fibers run roughly parallel to the edge of the vocal fold. From a mechanical point of view, this contracting

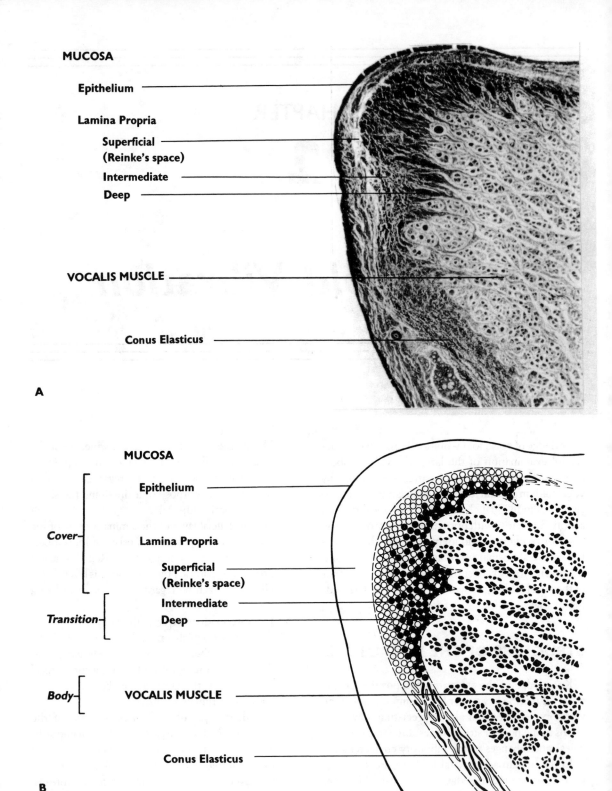

MUCOSA

Epithelium

Lamina Propria
Superficial
(Reinke's space)
Intermediate
Deep

VOCALIS MUSCLE

Conus Elasticus

A

MUCOSA

Epithelium

Cover

Lamina Propria
Superficial
(Reinke's space)
Intermediate
Transition Deep

Body **VOCALIS MUSCLE**

Conus Elasticus

B

Figure 2–1. A frontal section photo (A) and schematic (B) represent an adult human vocal fold through the middle of the membranous portion.

muscle is like a bundle of rather stiff rubber bands. The stiffness varies depending on the degree of contraction.

The border between the epithelium and the lamina propria is clear. The superficial layer of the lamina propria is also clearly delineated from the intermediate layer. There is, however, no clear-cut border between the intermediate and the deep layer of the lamina propria. As the vocalis muscle is approached, the number of elastic fibers decreases and that of collagenous fibers increases. Nor is the border between the lamina propria and the vocalis muscle clear either. Some collagenous fibers of the deep layer of the lamina propria insert deep into the muscle fiber bundles of the vocalis muscle.

The structure consisting of the intermediate and deep layers of the lamina propria is generally known as the vocal ligament. The vocal ligament is the uppermost portion of the conus elasticus. There is, however, a controversy in anatomical terminology with respect to this ligament. One camp of anatomists (Fujita & Fujita, 1981) includes the vocal ligament in the lamina propria; the other (Hirano, 1974) describes the vocal ligament as the tela submucosa. The vocal ligament is the uppermost portion of the conus elasticus. Fortunately, the terminology is not the important issue here.

What is important in this structure is that there are gradual changes in stiffness from the very pliable superficial layer of the lamina propria to the rather stiff vocalis muscle. Because differences in stiffness result in different mechanical properties and different mechanical properties have different vibration characteristics, it is important to consider this layered structure from a mechanical point of view. The five layers can be reclassified into three sections: the cover, consisting of the epithelium and the superficial layer of the lamina propria; the transition, consisting of the vocal ligament; and the body, consisting of the vocalis muscle. The mechanical properties of the cover and the transition are passively controlled by the laryngeal muscles, whereas those of the body are controlled actively by the muscle itself, as well as passively by the other laryngeal muscles.

Except for a few variations, the vocal fold is generally homogeneous along its length (Figure 2-2).

At the anterior commissure is a mass of collagenous fibers, referred to as the anterior commissure tendon, or Broyles tendon. It is a continuation of the inner thyroid perichondrium. Posterior to this is another mass, the anterior macula flava, consisting chiefly of elastic fibers and fibroblasts. It is a continuation of the intermediate layer of the lamina propria. Thus, changes in stiffness are gradual from the stiff thyroid cartilage to the pliable mucosa of the vocal fold. At the posterior end of the membranous portion of the vocal fold is another mass, the posterior macula flava, consisting chiefly of elastic fibers and fibroblasts. It is a variation of the intermediate layer of the lamina propria and attaches to the vocal process of the arytenoid cartilage with an intervening transitional structure. Here again, changes in stiffness are gradual between the stiff arytenoid cartilage and the pliable mucosa of the vocal fold. Variations of the structure occurring at both ends appear to be important for protection of the vocal fold from mechanical damage caused possibly by vibration.

The vocal fold structure changes as a function of age. In the vocal fold of human newborns (Figures 2-3 & 2-4), there is no vocal ligament and, therefore, the entire lamina propria of the mucosa is nearly uniform in structure. The elastic conus does not reach the vocal fold edge to form a ligament. Near the anterior and posterior ends are aggregations of fibers that are immature maculae flavae. From the mechanical point of view, one can postulate a two-layer vibratory structure consisting of the cover — for example, the entire mucosa — and the body — in another word, the muscle. The development of the layer structure is completed by the end of adolescence.

An important element of the layer structure is an additional layer outside the vocal fold — a layer of mucus, or a mucus blanket. Without this layer, in other words, if the vocal fold surface is completely dry, the vocal fold cannot vibrate (Hiroto, 1966). Mucus is not created at the edge of the membranous vocal fold, for no glands are located there. Rather, mucus (strictly speaking, mucoserous secretion) comes from the glands located superiorly, inferiorly, anteriorly, and posteriorly to the edge of the membranous vocal fold (Figure 2-5).

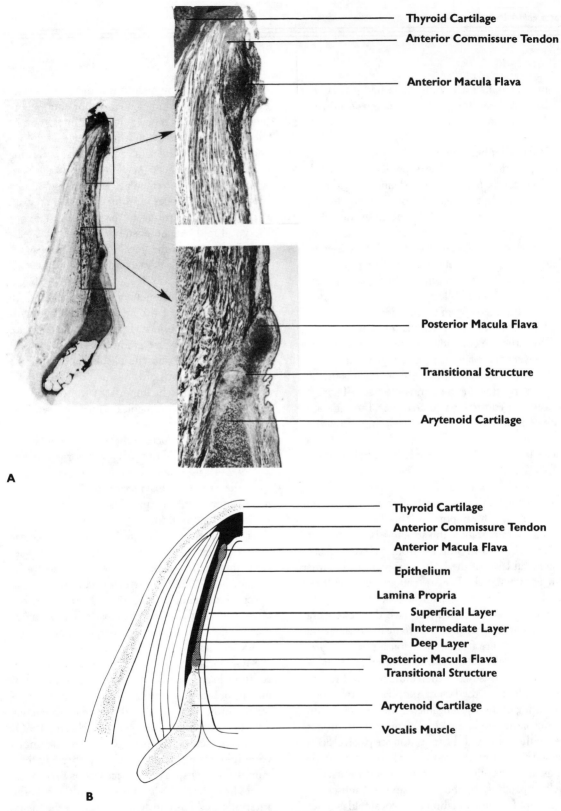

Figure 2-2. A horizontal section photo (A) and schematic (B) represent a human vocal fold edge.

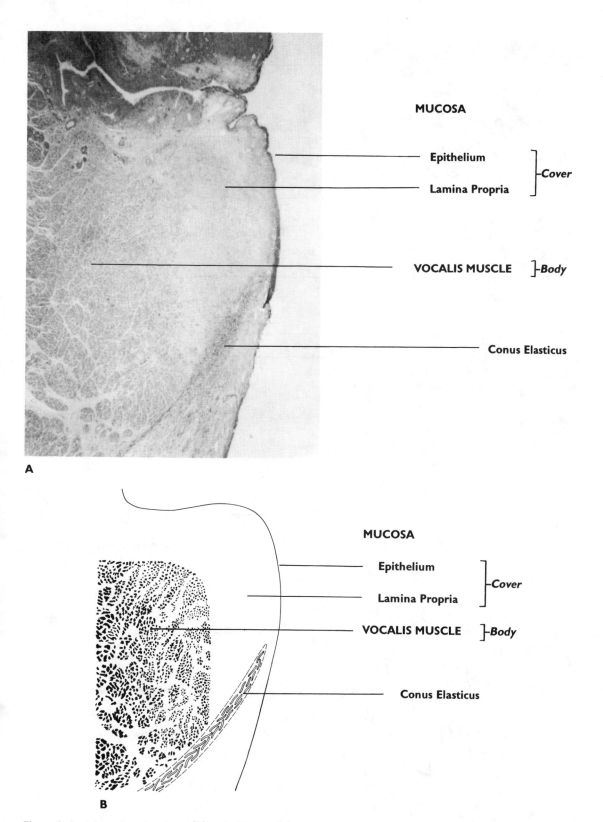

Figure 2–3. A frontal section photo (A) and schematic (B) represent a newborn vocal fold through the middle of the membraneous portion.

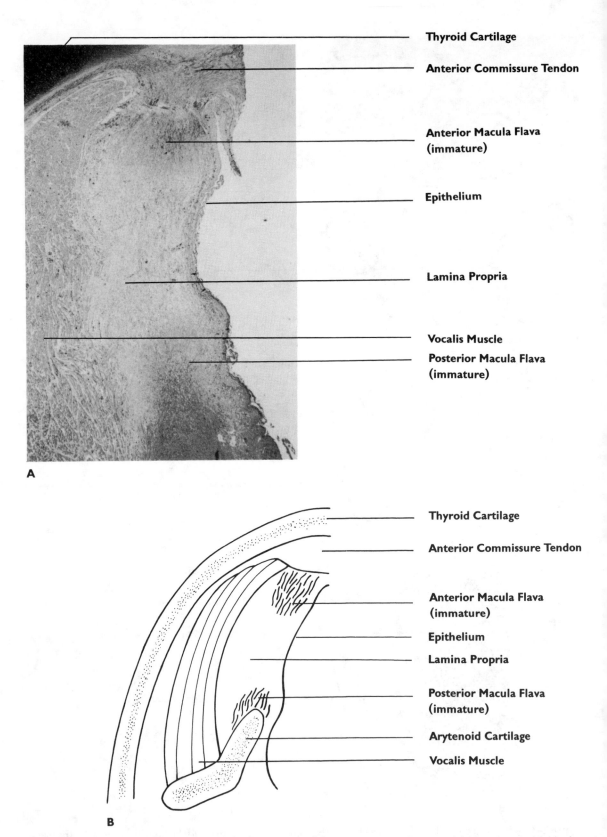

Figure 2-4. A horizontal section photo (A) and schematic (B) represent a newborn vocal fold at the vocal fold edge.

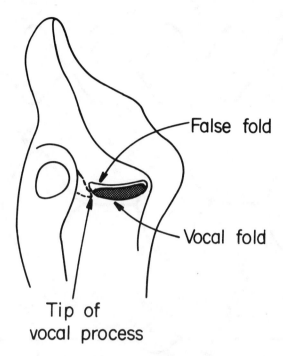

Figure 2–5. The glandless area (shadowed) of the larynx shown in schematic.

VIBRATORY PATTERNS

General Pattern

Normal vocal folds present three typical vibratory patterns: for falsetto, modal voice, and vocal fry (Figure 2–6). In the falsetto (light voice, or loft voice), no complete glottic closure takes place (Open Quotient = 1). Falsetto is usually associated with a high fundamental frequency. The modal voice (heavy voice), is associated with a complete glottic closure (Open Quotient < 1). It covers the major middle frequency range (approximately 100–300 Hz). In vocal fry (creaky voice), the closed phase is long relative to the entire period, and there are occasionally two open phases during one vibratory cycle (Moore & von Leden, 1958). Vocal fry is associated with very low fundamental frequency (approximately 30–75 Hz).

Figure 2–7 schematically shows the behavior of the vocal fold in one vibratory cycle for modal voice. Because the vocal fold consists of multiple layers, each with different mechanical properties, the vibratory behavior differs from layer to layer. In the diagrams, the multiple-layer structure is simplified into a two-layer structure consisting of the pliable cover (the mucosa) and the rather stiff body (the muscle).

As the subglottal pressure increases against the closed glottis, the bilateral vocal folds are blown apart and the glottis opens. The vocal folds keep moving laterally until the subglottal pressure drops to a specific level. At the maximum opening, the upper part of the vocal fold edge (the so-called "upper lip") keeps moving laterally while the lower part of the edge (the so-called "lower lip") is moving medially. At a certain point in time, the upper lip also begins moving medially.

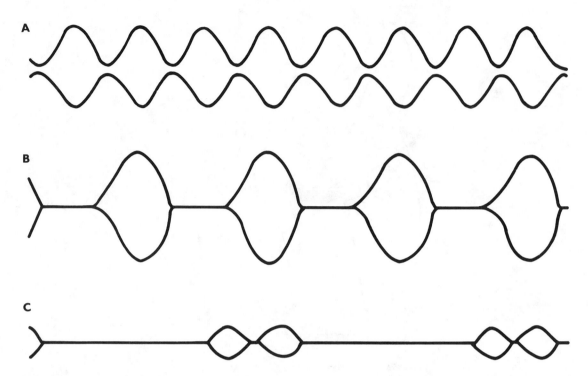

Figure 2–6. Vibratory patterns of normal vocal folds (modified from Hirano, 1981a) are typical for the falsetto (A), modal (B), and fry (C) voice.

Initially, the medial movement of the vocal folds results primarily from the recoiling force. As the vocal folds approach each other, narrowing the glottis, a negative pressure caused by the Bernoulli effect is built up in the glottis. This negative pressure sucks the vocal folds into close contact. The contact usually takes place first at the lower lip of the edge of the vocal folds. The contact area of the vocal fold increases until the subglottic pressure becomes high enough to blow apart the vocal folds. This aeromechanical action is repeated and results in phonation.

One of the most important features in vocal fold vibration is the occurrence of waves travelling on the mucosa from the inferior to superior surface of the vocal fold. These are referred to as mucosal waves. Not fixed landmarks of the vocal folds, but rather peaks that are identifiable in a specific phase during vibration, these waves change location with the vi-

bratory movements. The existence of a pliable mucosa is essential to the occurrence of the mucosal wave.

Parameters to Describe Vibratory Patterns

Certain phonatory features and concepts, when taken together, characterize the voice. The clinician who understands these phenomena can appreciate their value when interpreting the subjective visible perceptual ratings of videostroboscopic vibratory patterns.

The first is fundamental frequency, the basic frequency of the voice. The time span required for one entire vibratory cycle is called the fundamental period. Cycle-to-cycle variations of the fundamental period normally occur. The fundamental

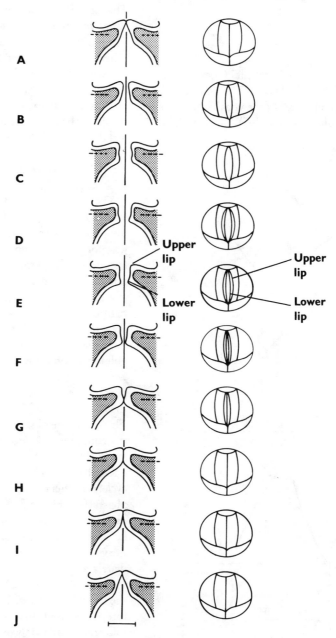

A

B

C

D

Upper
lip

Upper
lip

E

Lower
lip

Lower
lip

F

G

H

I

J

Figure 2–7. In schematic, simplified, mucosa and muscle presentation of vocal fold vibration the left column offers a frontal section of the vocal fold for modal voice and the right column, a view from above (modified from Hirano, 1981a).

frequency (F_o) and the fundamental period (P) are related as:

$$F_o \times P = 1$$

Another major feature is horizontal (latero-medial) excursion of the vocal fold edge. The term "edge" refers to the observable part of the vocal fold that is located most medially (Figure 2–7). During vibra-

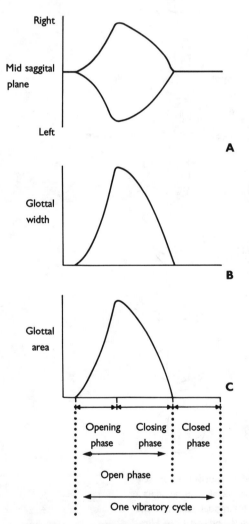

Figure 2–8. Phases describe one vibratory cycle: A, Horizontal excursion; B, Glottal width; and C, Glottal area (modified from Hirano, 1981a).

tion, the edge is not a fixed part of the vocal fold. The observable innermost part of the vocal fold varies within each vibratory cycle (see Figure 2–7). The horizontal edge serves as a landmark from which other observations of amplitude changes and extent of closure can be made. The edge of the vocal fold also moves in vertical and longitudinal directions, but it is difficult to quantify the movements in these directions by observing from above. The latero-medial displacement of the vocal folds is called amplitude. Amplitude normally varies a bit from cycle to cycle. The distance between the edges of the vocal folds is called "glottal width."

The area surrounded by the edges of the vocal folds is called the glottal area. In normal vibrations, the glottal area waveform resembles the glottal width waveform as determined at the point of the greatest excursion. The glottal area waveform is similar but not identical to the volume velocity waveform. Usually, the volume velocity waveform is skewed to the right of the glottal area waveform. The degree of a skewing depends on the shape of the vocal tract, force of glottal closure, duration of open phase, and pulmonary pressure.

One vibratory cycle is divided into two major phases: open and closed. During the closed phase, the contact area of the bilateral vocal folds changes. This cannot be observed from above. The nature of the contact area is revealed through electroglottography (EGG) and/or ultrasound glottography. The open phase, which occupies the greatest part of the cycle, is further divided into the opening and closing phases (see Figure 2–8). At certain phases during each vibratory cycle, two eminences — the "upper lip" and "lower lip" — are observed near the edge of the vocal fold. They are usually best observed immediately after maximum opening of the vocal folds (see Figure 2–7 D, E, F). During the opening phase, the lower lip is covered by the upper lip and, therefore, is not visible from above. The edge of the vocal fold represents mainly the upper lip. During the closing phase, the two lips are usually observable from above. The closed phase typically begins with an approximation of the lower lips. The edge of the vocal fold, therefore, represents mainly the lower lip during the closing phase. In the closed phase, the upper and lower lips become indistinguishable.

It is important to stress that the upper and lower lips are not definite portions of a vocal fold. The locations of these eminences vary with time within each vibratory cycle.

The open phase, with its two phases — opening and closing — is used to compute glottal area function measures, open quotient (OQ), speed quotient (SQ) and speed index (SI).

The open quotient is defined as:

$$OQ = \frac{t \text{ (open phase)}}{t \text{ (entire phase)}}$$

where t = time.

The longer the open phase is, the larger is the OQ. OQ = 1 when there is no complete glottal closure.

The speed quotient (SQ) is defined as:

$$SQ = \frac{t \text{ (opening phase)}}{t \text{ (closing phase)}} = \frac{\text{average speed of closing}}{\text{average speed of opening}}$$

where t = time.

If SQ < 1, then the closing takes longer than the opening; if the SQ > 1, the opening takes longer than the closing.

The speed index (SI) is defined (Hirano, 1974) as:

$$SI = \frac{t \text{ (opening phase)} - t \text{ (closing phase)}}{t \text{ (opening phase)} + t \text{ (closing phase)}} = \frac{SQ - 1}{SQ + 1}$$

Figure 2–9 represents the relationship between SQ and SI. SI seems to be a better measure than SQ, and to relate more to our intuitive sense of scaling, for several reasons: (1) SI ranges only from −1 to 1 whereas SQ ranges over infinitely large values (0 to ∞); (2) when two waveforms have the same triangular shape and one is the reverse of the other (with respect to time), SI takes equal absolute values with reverse signs (see Figure 2–9), whereas SQ takes two different values whose product is 1; (3) one can visualize the waveform from SI values more easily than from SQ values; and (4) SI has a more direct rela-

tionship with the spectral characteristics of the waveform than does SQ.

The mucosal wave is another significant feature. In the normal vocal fold, waves travelling on the mucosa from the inferior to the superior surface are observed during phonation, except for falsetto. The speed of the wave is normally 0.5 to 1 m/sec. Existence of a soft and pliant superficial layer of the lamina propria is essential for the occurrence of the mucosal wave.

A final important feature is that the structure of the normal vocal fold is generally homogeneous along its longitudinal axis. Individual points along the longitudinal axis do not usually present substantial phase differences. The amplitude is usually greatest near the middle portion of the membranous part of the vocal fold.

Symmetry of the vibratory movement of the vocal folds is another major feature. Symmetrical movement indicates that their mechanical properties are the same. Differences in mechanical properties of the two vocal folds result in asymmetrical vibrations.

METHODS OF EXAMINATION OF VOCAL FOLD VIBRATION

The vocal folds usually vibrate at 100–300 Hz during normal conversation, and at 1000 Hz or higher during singing. Observation of such vibrations cannot be made with the naked eye and requires special techniques. Of the six methods currently available — stroboscopy, X-ray stroboscopy, ultra-high-speed photography, photoelectric glottography, electroglottography, and ultrasound glottography — stroboscopy is the most useful for clinical purposes.

Ultra-high-speed photography has been employed chiefly for research and educational purposes, but the apparatus is too expensive, and the data processing is too time-consuming for most clinicians. With ultra-high-speed photography, views from above are available, but the status below the glottis is not visualized. This is a limitation of stroboscopy, too, but its other advantages render this a less vital concern for stroboscopy.

Glottographies provide some information about vocal fold vibration, but the vibration of the vocal fold itself is not directly viewed.

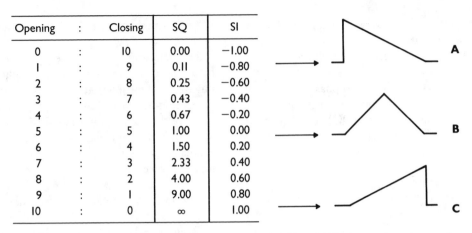

Opening	:	Closing	SQ	SI
0	:	10	0.00	−1.00
1	:	9	0.11	−0.80
2	:	8	0.25	−0.60
3	:	7	0.43	−0.40
4	:	6	0.67	−0.20
5	:	5	1.00	0.00
6	:	4	1.50	0.20
7	:	3	2.33	0.40
8	:	2	4.00	0.60
9	:	1	9.00	0.80
10	:	0	∞	1.00

Figure 2–9. Waveforms illustrate speed indices for −1.00, 0.00, and 1.00, showing how the opening and closing phases and SQ co-vary.

In photoelectric glottography (PGG), the glottal area variation is recorded with the use of a photoelectric device that converts light intensity into electric voltage. The glottis is illuminated from above or below with DC light and the intensity of light passing through the glottis is measured with a sensor placed on the opposite side. Photoelectric glottography gives some information during open phase. Some problems exist with the validity of the quantitative information obtained from photoelectric glottography.

EGG measures the electrical impedance between two electrodes placed above the thyroid laminae. The signal reflects contact area between the two vocal folds, but interpretation of EGG waveform appears to be controversial, especially in pathological cases. When electroglottograms are obtained concurrently with other recordings of vocal fold vibration, the interpretation of EGG becomes more reliable.

In ultrasound glottography, the border between the vocal fold surface and the air in the glottis is determined on the basis of the difference in acoustic impedance between the two media. Ultrasound glottography gives some information during both open and closed phases. Space resolution of ultrasound glottograms is not very high.

A great advantage of glottographies is that immediate graphic displays of the results can be obtained. However, neither the vibratory behavior of each vocal fold nor that of different portions of each vocal fold can be evaluated by means of glottographies. These can be observed only with stroboscopy and ultra-high-speed photography. This information is the most relevant from a clinical point of view.

Videostroboscopy offers affordability, ease of use, and a permanent record of perceptions. Moreover, it allows the clinician to capture movement so it can be quantitatively and qualitatively rated and compared with other data within and between patients, pathologies, treatments, and programs, and even from other examining technologies.

This ability to characterize the vocal fold vibrations is a product of the appropriate instrumentation and operation of the videostroboscopic equipment.

STUDY QUESTIONS

1. The area in which a vocal fold lesion will make the greatest perceptual difference in voice production is:

   a. Reinke's space.

   b. Epithelium.

   c. The layers of the lamina propria.

   d. The vocalis muscle.

   e. All of the above.

2. The layer of the lamina propria that consists primarily of loose fibers and matrix is:

   a. Not very pliable.

   b. The intermediate layer.

   c. Contains the vocalis muscle.

   d. Considered Reinke's space, the superficial layer.

3. The structure consisting of the intermediate and deep layers of the lamina propria is generally known as:

   a. The vocalis muscle.

   b. The vocal ligament.

   c. The false fold.

   d. The glottis.

4. The five layers of the vocal fold structure are divided into three sections. The first section, the cover, consists of the epithelium and:

   a. The superficial layer of the lamina propria.

   b. The vocalis muscle.

   c. Mucosa.

   d. The vocal ligament.

5. The important component of the histological structure of the vocal fold is:

   a. The varying thicknesses.

   b. The body-cover relationship.

   c. The gradual changes in stiffness throughout structure.

   d. The rocking motion of the cricoid and the thyroid cartilages.

   e. None of the above.

6. Vocal fold structure changes as a function of age. The main histological difference in the vocal fold of a newborn versus that of an adolescent is:

   a. There is no anterior commissure.

   b. The arytenoids are fixed.

   c. There is no "transition" or vocal ligament.

   d. The layers are very thick to withstand the excessive crying.

7. Without this component outside the vocal fold, vibration of the folds cannot occur:

   a. Sensory fibers.

   b. A layer of mucus.

   c. Mucus glands at the edge of the vocal fold.

   d. Subglottic pressure.

8. There are three typical vibratory patterns: falsetto, modal, and vocal fry. The pattern used during conversational speech would be:

   a. Falsetto.

   b. Modal and vocal fry.

   c. Falsetto and vocal fry.

   d. Modal.

9. The force that moves the vocal folds to a medial position is:

   a. Gravity.

   b. Subglottic pressure.

   c. The Bernoulli effect.

   d. The Doppler effect.

10. One of the most important features to look for when viewing vocal fold vibration is:

   a. Uniformity of the arytenoids.

   b. The mucosal wave.

   c. The perioral sinuses.

   d. The glottis

11. The parameter(s) to be tuned into when viewing videostroboscopic vibratory patterns is (are):

   a. Fundamental frequency.

   b. Latero-medial excursion of the vocal fold edge.

   c. Mucosal wave.

   d. Homogeneity and symmetry of the vocal fold.

   e. All of the above.

12. Which of the following methods would be most useful for clinical viewing of vocal fold vibration?

   a. Ultra-high-speed photography.

   b. Stroboscopy.

   c. Electroglottography.

   d. X-ray stroboscopy.

CHAPTER

3

Instrumentation and Operation

Stroboscopy, coupled with endoscopes and video recording equipment, has revolutionized the diagnosis and treatment of voice disorders. As the recorded data are of a true image of the vocal fold, the viewer has direct access to the vibratory pattern and does not have to infer what is happening from peripheral measures.

Reports on the clinical utility of stroboscopy are abundant (Alberti, 1978; Faure & Muller, 1992; Hirano, 1981a, 1988; Wendler, 1992). These reports have established the value of stroboscopy in the assessment and evaluation of treatment of voice disorders: One can observe hyperfunction of the larynx; changes in stiffness resulting from laryngeal carcinoma, papilloma, or scar tissue; passive movement of paralyzed vocal folds; asymmetries of vibration; and effects of vocal fold edema on the vibratory pattern of the larynx.

Such observations are possible with good instrumentation and proper operation of the equipment and conduct of the videostroboscopic examination. Implementing these clinical assessment procedures depends on the type of equipment, the examiner's skills and the patient's needs, the goal of image quality, and the ever-present health concerns of any medical procedure.

BASIC INSTRUMENTATION

Stroboscopes

Many different kinds of stroboscopes and auxiliary equipment are available for stroboscopic examinations of the larynx (Figures 3-1 & 3-2). The basic equipment consists of a microphone, light source, electronic control unit, and foot pedal. The microphone, which is applied to the patient's neck just below the larynx, is used to trigger the stroboscopic light source; it directs the sound waves to the electronic control unit for filtration and amplification. The control unit transmits the extracted fundamental period of the voice signal to a xenon lamp that emits an intermittent beam of white light pulses synchronous with the voice signal, varies the phase point with the light flashes, and indicates the fun-

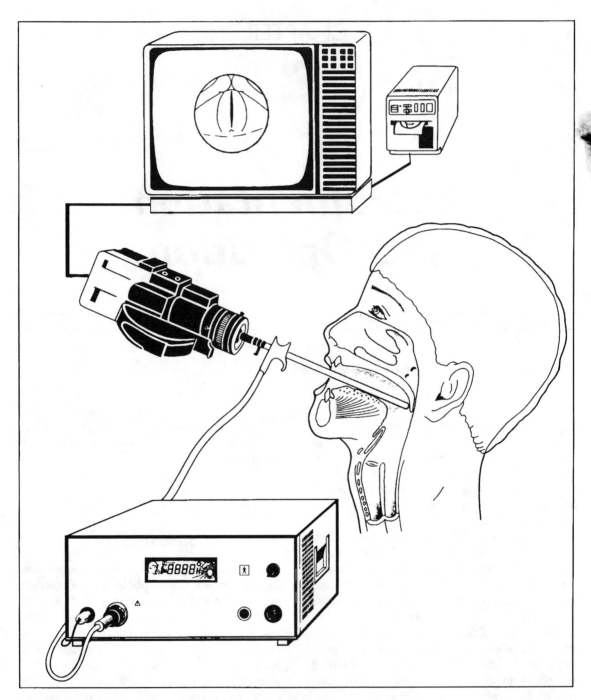

Figure 3–1. Pictured is a Brüel and Kjaer Stroboscopic system illustrating the main components of the system.

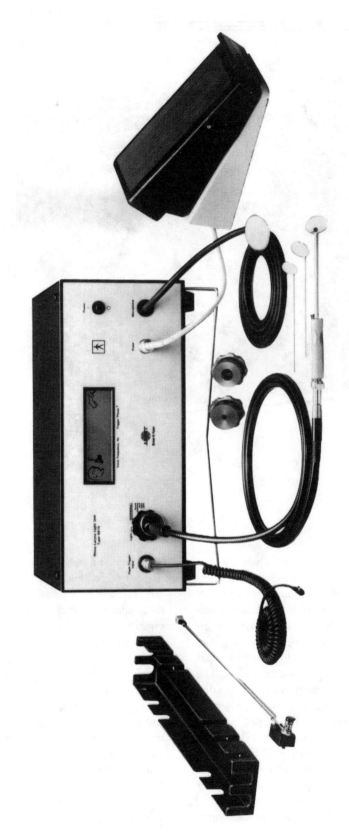

A

Figure 3–2. (A) photograph of the Bruel & Kjaer stroboscope and (B) photograph of the Storz stroboscope (on following page).

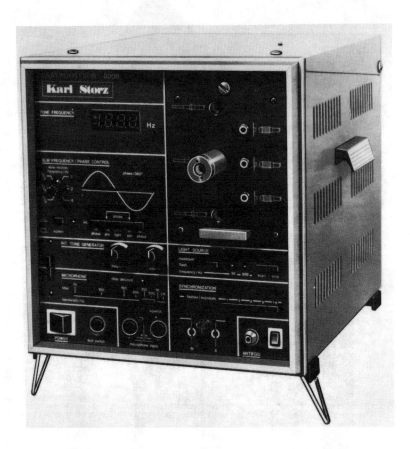

Figure 3–2. B

damental frequency of phonation. Thus, the frequency of the light flashes corresponds to the frequency of the vocal fold vibrations, regardless of pitch or pitch change, unless the flash rate is modified by the examiner. The pulsed light beam is directed by an operating microscope, an ordinary head mirror, or by light cables and endoscope to the larynx, as in any indirect laryngoscopic procedure. The stroboscopic view of the larynx can be recorded from a laryngeal mirror, a rigid endoscope, a flexible endoscope, or an operating microscope.

Using a stroboscopic light (see Figure 3–3) with an ordinary operating microscope (focal distance to objective < 40 μm) provides a magnification of 6X when the image is seen in the laryngeal mirror (Fex & Elmqvist, 1973; McKelvie, Grey, & North, 1970). Operating microscopes have excellent optic

resolution and stereoscopic sight, can provide a permanent record with unequaled detail of the structure, and can provide an accurate means of making measurements, which cannot be done by the other visualization techniques.

Several auxiliary features are built into most stroboscopic systems. An auxiliary observation light system provides illumination of the larynx with a constant light source during respiration and other nonphonatory tasks. This light is usually brighter, and provides better images and more accurate representation of color. Meters or digital readouts on the stroboscope or video monitor indicate the F_o being produced. Some stroboscopes also indicate the phonation intensity level. The frequency of light flashes can be controlled by the examiner using either a foot pedal or a switch. This permits a change

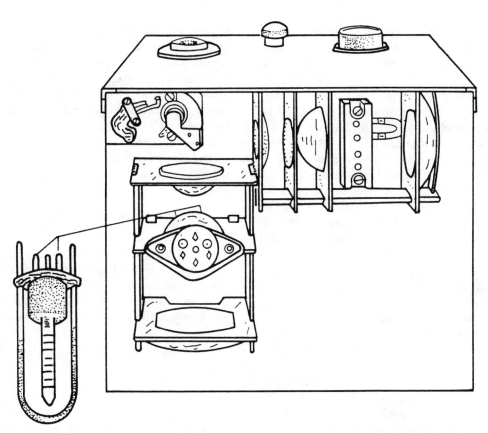

Figure 3-3. An interior view of the inside of a typical stroboscope illustrates the stroboscopic light source. This xenon lamp is first charged by a power supply and then discharged in approximately 1/1000 second through an inert gas contained in the bulb. The bulb should not be touched by fingers because of the oil residue they leave on the surface. The orientation to the mirror reflector is critical in getting optimal light. The light must be centered relative to the reflector and in close proximity.

in the phase angle of the light flashes in relation to the sound impulses to obtain either a stationary image of the vocal folds at any instant of the vibration or the typical slow-motion effect.

A 35mm or video camera can be connected to the eyepiece of a rigid endoscope, a fiberscope, or an operating microscope. For high quality fiberscopic recordings, it is essential that the cameras are sensitive to light levels below 7 lux, with a somewhat higher level (10 lux) tolerated if recordings are to be made with a rigid endoscope. In all areas concerned with optics (cameras, recorders, endoscopes), the technology is changing so rapidly that anything written today might be dated tomorrow. (For further readings on the basics of lens and video technology see Selkin, 1983a, b; Wilson, Kudryk, & Sych, 1986; Yanagihara, 1967). Good recordings can currently be obtained from some of the inexpensive color video camera recording systems designed for home use or for surveillance.

Light Source

The light output needs to be bright enough to be used with flexible fiberscopes and render good video images. In fiberscopes, light is concentrated in a beam transmitted via light-carrying cables to illuminate the larynx. Some fiberscopes' light-carrying bundles can lose 60–90% of the available light.

Light has a frequency at which it will maximally perform with one pulse per cycle. If the selected frequency is too high, recordings for males will be poor; conversely, if the selected frequency is too low, children and sopranos might not be recorded well. The light is coupled to lenses and mirrors to maximize its reflection. Longer pulses produce brighter light, but also can blur the image when motion occurs within the time frame of the pulse.

Whereas other light bulbs appear to burn out instantaneously, the stroboscopic light burns down and provides progressively less illumination. Because this process is gradual, it can go undetected until the clinician happens to compare recordings made over a time span. The difference can be dramatic. One way to keep this in check is to install a light-calibrating box. A calibration box is one means of monitoring the degradation of illumination of the stroboscopic light.

It is possible to build a light-calibrating box by lining a shoe box completely with black felt. The floor of the box is mounted with a colored strip that should include red, blue, and white. The strip of colors featured on most videotape cartons works well for this purpose. A small hole, just large enough to accommodate the endoscope is cut in one end. The endoscope is inserted perpendicular to the bottom of the box. A recording of the color bar is made with each new strobe light, and the recording is saved for reference. A second tape is used for the actual examination recordings. As the light diminishes, direct comparisons of the two tapes will reveal that the image becomes darker. Obviously, this diagnosis presumes that all other parts of the system are functioning properly.

Endoscopes

Selection of endoscopes depends on the population being studied and the need to obtain connected speech versus sustained vowel production. The flexible endoscope permits assessment of velopharyngeal function without inhibiting movement of the oral structures. It also allows for examination of gross arytenoid movement during whistling and production of undistorted words and phrases by the patient. Karnell (1991) suggests that flexible scopes in the hands of experienced, skilled endoscopists minimizes the risk of triggering a gag reflex in the patient, a common problem encountered when oral laryngoscopes are used.

Rigid laryngoscopes, by contrast, provide increased illumination and magnified images relative to those obtained with flexible endoscopes.

OPERATION

Critical to the routine application of videostroboscopy is an understanding of potential pitfalls in the operation of the instrumentation and roles of the examiner and the patient. The clinic is not a laboratory in which all variables can be easily controlled.

Examiner's Knowledge

To use stroboscopy in a meaningful manner, the examiner must have knowledge of sound production and laryngeal pathology, skill with the technique, and ability to interpret the recordings.

Sound Production

Vocal fold vibration varies tremendously with sex, age, mode of phonation, respiratory support, anxiety, and so forth. For example, as vocal pitch increases, the vocal folds elongate, the mucosal wave is reduced, and glottal closure changes. Similarly when intensity is increased, changes in the vibratory pattern are also evident — the amplitude of vibration increases and the larynx is closed for a longer period. Failure to understand these influences on sound production can cause major problems when the examiner seeks to interpret the data. Because of these frequency-intensity interrelationships, it is crucial that examiners be aware of recording conditions and make quantitative measurements and perceptual judgments of quality at the time of the recording.

Normal variations in other parameters illustrate this point. The mucosal wave during normal pitch and loudness moves in a wave-like fashion, much like ripples when a stone is dropped in a pond. Absence or reduction of the mucosal wave can occur with many pathologies, including vocal fold edema and laryngeal carcinoma. Mucosal wave is also reduced with hyperfunction, which can occur in people who are anxious during the stroboscopic examination or who make an increased effort to comply with examiner instructions. Because the mucosal wave is also reduced during high-pitch productions, it is critical that the examiner note the type of phonation and frequency of production.

Laryngeal Pathology

Equally important to interpretation is the examiner's knowledge of normal anatomy and physiology, as well as differences related to sex. Clinicians must be familiar with what to expect for various pathologies and laryngeal disorders to get the best image possible to gain the best information for diagnostic decisions and for treatment monitoring. For instance, asymmetry of movement is one of the variables observed. When making judgments, the examiner should recognize that asymmetry is the rule rather than the exception and that laryngeal asymmetries appear to be exacerbated by age (Hirano, Yoshida, Yoshida, & Tateishi, 1987). The functional significance of these asymmetries is unknown, but it is clear that an asymmetrical larynx might not necessarily be the cause of a given presenting disorder.

Another parameter is aperiodicity. Aperiodicity is generally thought to result from an imbalance of muscular forces or unequal weighting of the right and left vocal folds. A common variation is aperiodicity at the end of lung volume or at the lower end of the pitch and loudness range. Like asymmetries, aperiodicity also appears to be exacerbated with age.

Normal variations in glottal closure occur with changes in pitch and loudness and with the sex of the speaker. A well-known variation in glottal closure relates to high-pitch production in which closure is incomplete. Male-female differences in glottic closure are less well-documented. For example, during normal pitch and loudness conditions, the majority of females have a glottal chink and appear, in general, to have a shorter closed phase than do

male counterparts. There are also sex differences associated with age: It is rare to see a geriatric female with vocal fold bowing, but common to see it in males in their senior years.

Obviously, if we are to really understand "normal variations," we need to have a large normal data base developed across age levels for males and females. However, in the absence of such, clinicians must be familiar with normal variations to differentiate the normal from the abnormal. Failure to consider normal variations in phonation can result in erroneously attributing reduced mucosal wave or incomplete closure to a pathology, when, in fact, it is due to normal differences in phonation related to age, sex, or phonatory condition.

Thus, examiner-related variables are not entirely independent of normal variations. Clearly, the quality and accuracy of the interpretations will be, to a large degree, determined by the training of the observer and his or her knowledge of the anatomical, physiological, and instrumental factors influencing quality of the video image.

Skill With Technique

Generally, the operation of the stroboscope and the examination are simple for both the examiner and the patient. Occasionally, problems occur with the equipment. Two problems the examiner can encounter are back strain and foot-pedal position. In the past, heavy cameras coupled to endoscopes were balanced on clinicians' shoulders. The weight, in addition to the somewhat contorted position of the examiner relative to the patient, reportedly resulted in strain and back pain that was relieved only by temporary cessation of the activity. Today, back strain is less likely to occur with the new silicon-chip cameras, which are small and lightweight. Nevertheless it is suggested that people with known back problems use a weighted pulley for holding the endoscope and camera, to relieve the examiner of the weight and the necessity of positioning his or her shoulder in an abnormal position, leaving the clinician free to merely guide equipment placement. It is also suggested that the examiner sit rather than stand. Occasionally, examiners wearing high heels find the foot pedal unwieldy (Figure 3–4), and, in

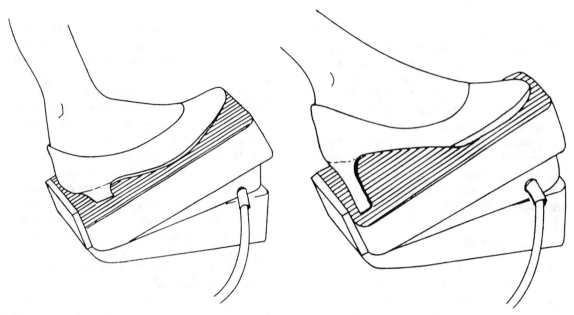

Figure 3-4. Depiction of source of postural difficulties associated with high heels and foot pedal operation. To counteract difficulties examiner can use a chair rather than stand, or wear flat shoes.

attempting to adjust to the unusual angle, place themselves in a position vulnerable to back strain.

Skill in Interpretation

Stroboscopic observations depend on subjective evaluations by the examiner. It is necessary for the examiner to practice rating normal and abnormal recordings if he or she is to make accurate observations of movement. Repeated observations of typical subjects of both sexes and all ages phonating at a variety of fundamental frequencies and intensities provide the examiner with a guide to normal variations. Viewing ultra-high-speed films of normal and pathological conditions is also extremely instructive.

Like auditory-perceptual judgments, visual perceptual judgments are likely to be influenced by observer bias (Teitler, 1992). Although the data on this topic are meager, there is considerable research on biases that influence other clinical judgments that might be relevant to stroboscopic ratings. Ramig (1975) has pointed out that "the expectation a person has when entering a situation not only accentuates what he will see, but also limits the likelihood of perceiving information contradictory to this expectancy" (p. 5). Lopez (1989) differentiates two types of bias. The first is called "overpathologizing" bias, by which a patient is perceived as more disturbed than he or she actually is, or as requiring more treatment than necessary. The other type is called "minimizing" bias, by which health personnel dismiss signs of organic disorders. Lopez (1989) argues that "this type of bias has consequences that may be as damaging to the patient as the overpathologizing bias may be; services are not rendered, even though there is a significant need for them" (p. 358). Observer bias needs to be taken into consideration when interpreting videostroboscopic images. Perceptual judgments are best accomplished with a checklist or rating scale. Even though the use of a rating scale and considerable practice in looking at normal and disordered larynges might help reduce bias (see Chapters 2, 5, & 6), it is unlikely that it would be totally eliminated.

Several scales have been developed and applied to the dysphonic population. Although similar in concept, each of the scales differs in the number of vocal features rated, the type of scale used (e.g., magnitude estimation, equal appearing interval, or paired comparisons), and the type and amount of listener training suggested. These differences and the lack of standards in perceptual testing make it nearly impossible to make interinstitutional comparisons. To reduce guesswork and observer bias, high-quality video recordings should be made, employing a standard test protocol specific to the disorder presented. The test protocol should include changes in pitch and loudness. For judgments to have any degree of reliability, it is necessary to have rigorous viewer training and recording standards — training and standards currently lacking in many clinical settings. When attempting to determine efficacy of treatment, examiners can make judgments by using a simple paired comparison in which he or she decides which of two samples looks better or by using a more elaborate rating scale in which the examiner rates each sample on a variety of different stroboscopic parameters. In routine clinic practice, stroboscopists generally rate a minimum of five parameters (symmetry of amplitude, phase of vibration, mucosal wave, periodicity, and glottal closure). More elaborate rating scales include observation of the vibrating edge, plane of approximation, and so on (see Appendix 3–1).

Patient Factors

Patient factors that affect videostroboscopic procedures include weak voice or inability to phonate at all, fear of the apparatus, hyperactive gag reflex, allergy to topical anesthetic, nasal polyps, or temporal mandibular joint problems (TMJ). When recognized before the examination begins, these problems are manageable.

If the patient's voice is too weak to activate the strobe, the driving force can be provided by placing the microphone on another speaker or by using a frequency oscillator. If the patient is totally aphonic, the stroboscopic light will not be a useful part of the examination, for no movement will be observed.

Use of the rigid endoscope can elicit gagging. Gagging should be avoided and might be best handled by one of two procedures. For the first, the patient is told that he or she may gag, and the procedure is briefly tried to test the patient's tolerance. Frequently patients tolerate it well, even when describing themselves as "wicked gaggers." If the patient can tolerate the procedure, the recording protocol is initiated; if not, a topical anesthesia is used. In extreme cases, tranquilizers can be given intravenously to diminish gagging. Others might better tolerate a flexible endoscope or the rigid endoscope after a conditioning program to enhance tolerance.

Some clinicians prefer to routinely apply topical anesthesia. Lidocaine® (Xylocaine 10% oral spray) acts on mucous membranes to produce local anesthesia by inhibiting the ionic fluxes required for the initiation and conduction of neural impulses. The anesthesia is rapid, occurring within 1–2 minutes and persisting for approximately 15 minutes. Lidocaine® is more rapidly absorbed in the presence of sepsis or traumatized mucosa. This is common and presents a strong rationale for the speech pathologist to administer this procedure only in a medically supervised setting where patient response can be monitored for any adverse effects and immediate treatment administered. Adverse side effects are usually dose-related and may result in CNS and cardiovascular system manifestations. Typical side effects include light-headedness, confusion or dizziness, and/or bradycardia or hypotension. Allergic reactions, including lesions, edema compromised airway, and anaphylactic reactions, are also possible.

Patients with a hyperactive gag reflex and allergies to topical anesthesia might be examined with the use of diazepam; often, neuroleptoanalgesia without intratracheal intubation is required to allow the subject to phonate with a laryngoscope in the throat; patients with nasal polyps generally do better with a rigid than a flexible endoscope. Patients with TMJ generally do better with a flexible as opposed to a rigid endoscope. When patients with TMJ are examined with a rigid endoscope, the protocol should be kept short to minimize the time the mouth must be open, and to decrease the probability of exacerbating mandibular muscle spasms.

Patient factors also affect the visual end product and data interpretation. These factors include the age of the patient, the anatomical structure, patient comfort, and examiner instructions and experience. In videostroboscopy, some imaging demands consideration of a series of compromises involving these factors to effect a useful and efficient examination. Each of these variables is affected by choices made regarding the type of endoscope to use, the field of view, and test tasks. Thus, protocol planning requires a clear understanding of the importance and influence of these multiple parameters on the final image.

In acoustic recording procedures, in which a standard protocol with a constant mouth-to-mike distance and speech tasks might be appropriate for all speakers, compromises involve the recording length. In stroboscopy, most compromises involve image acquisition. Some patients are not easily examined because anatomical features such as a subluxed arytenoid or omega-shaped epiglottis can obscure a view of the true vocal folds. Others might have large glottal gaps and concomitantly large losses of airflow making sustained phonatory tasks difficult, if not impossible. In some instances, such as in cases of spastic dysphonia, the examiner might want to have a large field of view to understand how the whole larynx operates in concert to produce the disordered voice, whereas, in others, such as in cases of infraglottal-level scar, the examiner might prefer a magnified view to determine how the scar impacts the vibratory pattern. Ideally, each patient would be examined during wide-angle field-of-view recordings and close-up magnifications recorded during a variety of phonatory tasks including both sustained phonation — produced at different pitch and loudness levels — and connected speech.

However, time is expensive and clinicians must be accountable to their patients and to their hospital administrators. Efficient patient care demands the maximum return for the amount of time invested in each imaging study. From the administrator's perspective, time is important because of the expense of laboratory equipment and the need to maintain a reasonable volume of patients. From the patient's perspective, time at a hospital is time away from work or home, and costly, unnecessary testing that does not provide unique information and that is done merely for knowledge's sake is unjustified. At any rate, the care and cooperation of the patient is integral to good videostroboscopic results, for, despite the smoothest procedures, visual perceptual judgments are complicated by issues in image quality.

IMAGE QUALITY

To be useful, a clinical image needs to provide adequate information to answer the clinical question being addressed. This then becomes the first requirement of image quality. In videostroboscopy, the image quality goal includes providing both an image that is clinically useful and an image that is aesthetically pleasing. This goal is most likely to be met if the image fills the monitor, if the vibratory edge can be easily visualized, if the mucosal wave can be visualized, if artifacts are minimized or absent, and if the processing and recording of the images are done carefully (Figure 3–5).

Artifacts

It is necessary to have a clear understanding of how artifacts arise and how extraneous factors can be controlled to ensure the best interpretation of results. Two major forms of artifacts are optical distortion and apparent motion. Placement of the endoscope and quality of the equipment have a major impact on optical distortion, and the distortion itself can actually create illusions of movement.

Optical Distortion

Optical distortions can arise from several factors: Endoscope placement can create the illusion of movement or of immobility and a false impression of size or location of lesions (even mucous can mimic a lesion in distant images as illustrated in Figure 3–6); and, pitch tracking problems can make the vocal folds appear to be moving or immobile when they are not. Consequently, any clinician attempting to provide objective documentation should be aware of potential artifacts.

Endoscope Placement. It has been well-documented that fiberoptic endoscopes are associated

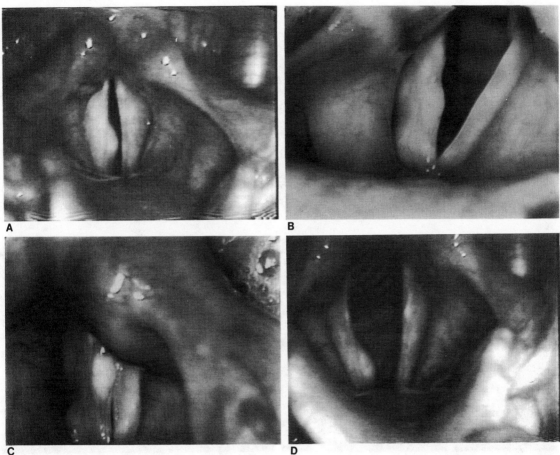

Figure 3–5. Video prints illustrating the ideal image filling the entire screen and different qualities related to differences in resolution of the video systems. (A) Image has good clarity but several bright spots where light is too intense. (B) Image is good and well focused. (C) Magnification is inadequate to visualize small changes, such as small hemorrhage. (D) Images are too dark.

with some optical distortion. Overall distortion of the resultant image can be divided into two categories: one related to the lens system of the fiberscope and the other related to the angle of the field of view axis and the distance of the fiberscope tip from the object. The former, a so-called "barrel-shaped" distortion, is independent of the lens-object angle and distance. In contrast, the latter *does* vary with those parameters.

Hibi, Bless, Hirano, and Yoshida (1988) report that the optical distortion related to lens-object angles and lens-object distances introduced by

flexible endoscopic examinations is systematic. The distortion can, therefore, be corrected through computer processing of the calibration input. The calibration and correction process is elaborate, expensive, and time-consuming, and, therefore, not clinically practical. Peppard and Bless (1989) suggest a simple, inexpensive procedure for making comparisons from recordings made at different times. Figure 3–7 illustrates this procedure. They suggest that clinicians use an overhead transparency placed on the video monitor to record and trace the placement of the laryngeal image. The traced image is

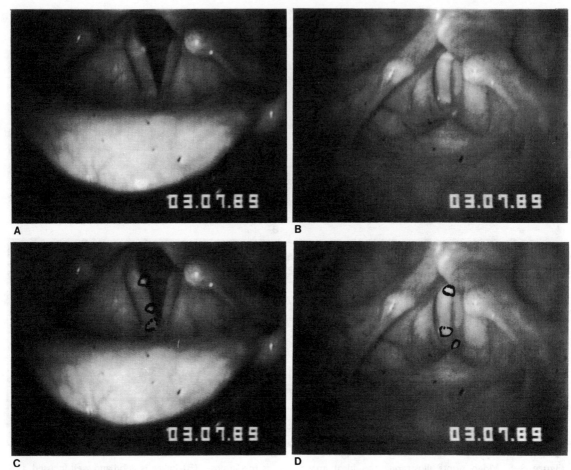

Figure 3-6. Mucus mimicking a lesion. Mucus is outlined in black in images C and D. Images A and B are untouched and illustrate how they might appear to be something else.

stored in the patient's chart. When the patient returns for the comparison recording, the transparency is placed on the screen, and the endoscopist positions the scope to produce nearly identical images. The inexpensive procedure adds only a couple of minutes to the examination and results in recordings that are comparable.

Another distortion problem is demonstrated by Casper, Brewer, and Colton (1987), who show that when one end of the endoscope is closer to the object being visualized than is the other, parallel lines appear to be in a V formation; one arytenoid will appear to be immobile or to move sluggishly relative to the contralateral side; and, in the case of bilateral lesions, the lesion closer to the lens will appear larger. This work underscores the need to create a nearly distortion-free image. This is achieved by placing the endoscope perpendicular to the floor and parallel to the superior surface of the larynx and in a position to center the image on the screen. The problem also underscores the need to execute every examination in as consistent a manner as is clinically feasible. Without correcting for lens-object angle and distance distortions, endoscopists cannot accurately measure glottal dimensions or the size of a lesion, and might, in fact, introduce foreshortening and/or elongation that would contribute to erroneous judgments about the

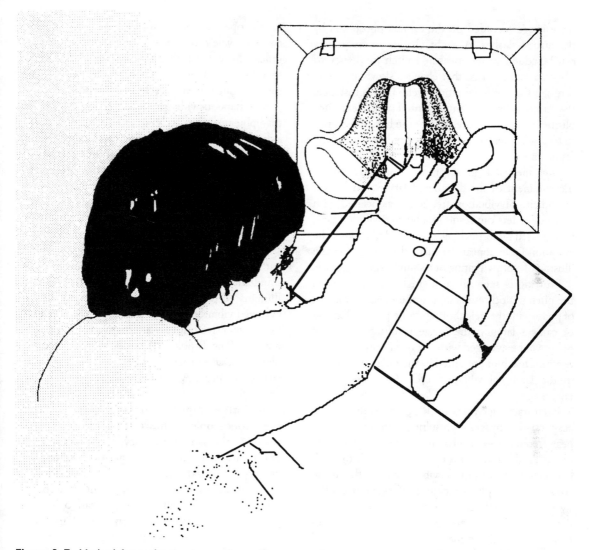

Figure 3–7. Method for replicating images for making pre- and post-treatment comparisons.

size and site of lesions and movement patterns of the larynx.

Pitch Tracking. A crucial part of the stroboscope instrument is the pitch-tracking circuit. The pitch-tracking circuit synchronizes the strobe flashes with the laryngeal vibration cycle to obtain a stable video image. This circuit needs to operate in real time across a multioctave pitch range. Any deficien-

cies in the performance of the pitch-tracking circuit will be reflected in degraded video images.

If the pitch-tracking circuit is functioning properly, the strobe pulses occur at a constant phase in the laryngeal vibration cycle, and a stable image of the larynx at the phase will result — provided the video camera phosphor latency is longer than the video frame interval. The video frame rate is not important here because each video frame "sees" the same image recorded on the camera phosphors by the strobe flashes. A slight change in frequency can be added to the measured pitch frequency to obtain a video image that changes slowly in phase through the entire vibration cycle. In this instance, the latency become important. For a clear, unblurred image, it is necessary for the hertz difference to be low compared to the phosphor latency and the frame rate.

Pitch measurement errors are more likely in the measurement of the disordered larynx. The lower periodicity of vibration frequently associated with voice disorders can result in a blurred video image, in increased pitch-tracking errors, and in making the vibration cycle appear irregular, thereby giving the illusion of a nonvibrating or a shimmering structure.

Blurring is seen when a single frame error in the pitch period results in a strobe pulse that is out of phase with the neighboring strobe pulses. Because of camera latency, the image resulting from this pulse will be averaged with the neighboring images, resulting in a blur presented by the phase differences in the laryngeal vibration cycle for these different images.

Pitch-tracking errors can change the order of successive video images — resulting from the use of a beat frequency — from that of linearly increasing phase. At this point, it is not possible to distinguish between irregularity of the vibration cycle that is the consequence of pitch-tracking artifact and irregularity that is directly connected with the disordered condition, without making simultaneous measurements of the audio signal or EGG. Thus, rapid and accurate tracking of the pitch is an essential component of the stroboscopic light and simultaneous measures of cycle-to-cycle variation essential to interpretation (Karnell, 1989, 1991; Sercarz, Berke, Gerratt, Kreiman, Ming, & Navidad, 1992; Sercarz, Berke, Ming, Gerratt, & Navidad, 1992).

Apparent Motion and Aperiodic Vibration

Unlike high-speed photography, which provides detailed information about each cycle of vibration, videostroboscopy, as previously stated, produces an optical illusion from optical fusion of several fragments of different cycles. True information concerning the opening and closing pattern variations from cycle to cycle can be lost in the averaging process, unless the videostroboscopic apparatus is coupled to other instruments — such as the EGG — that can account for each cycle of vibration.

Simultaneous videostroboscopic and electroglottographic recording techniques have been described as both inexpensive and technically simple (Karnell, 1991). The stroboscopic light source triggers an oscilloscope used to display the electroglottographic waveform. Each pulse produced by the stroboscope triggers an excursion of the oscilloscope beam across the display screen, so that the onset point of the beam excursion relates in time to the flash of the strobe light from the light source. Both the illuminated laryngeal image and the EGG waveform are simultaneously displayed on a split-screen video. Illuminated points are visually fused, providing an averaged vibratory pattern over successive cycles. A more expensive but easy alternative is the Kay Elemetrics (Pine Brook, NJ) stroboscope, which displays the EGG image on the video screen with the laryngeal image. An example is provided in Figure 3–8.

To further capitalize on optical phenomena, the stroboscopic flashes can be emitted in two ways: At the same frequency as phonation (synchronization) or at a slight variation of frequency (asynchronization).

Synchronization results in apparent "freezing" of the vocal folds. This allows the clinician to view any position to investigate the structure of the vocal folds and to determine if aperiodic vibration is occurring. Because the synchronized flashes should illuminate the same portion of the cycle for each flash, the vocal folds with periodic vibration should appear to stand still. In instances when movement is observable, the clinician can assume the presence of aperiodicity in the vocal fold vibration. Thus, folds that appear to shimmer or to continue moving under synchronized stroboscopic light indicate aperiodic vibration.

By contrast, asynchronization — with a slight variation between the frequency of pulses of illumination and the frequency of the sound being phonated — will cause normal vocal folds to appear to move in slow motion (see Chapter 2).

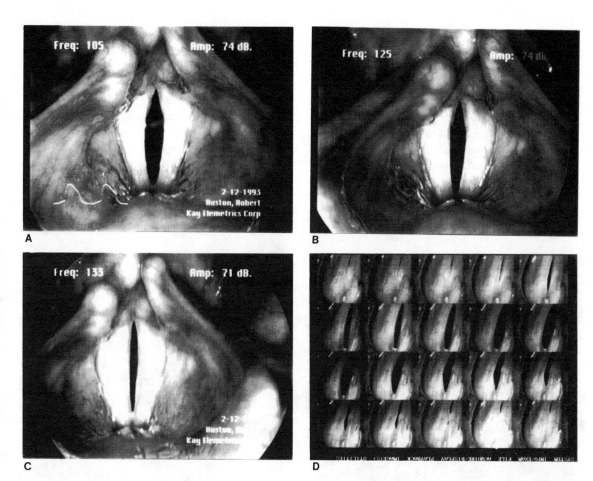

Figure 3–8. (A, B, C) These sharp, clear images show changes in amplitude of movement. The amplitude (distance of glottal edge from midline) is great in A, normal in B, and small in C, as one might see in high-frequency productions. (D) The composite illustrates how amplitude changes across vibratory cycles from nearly complete closure to a large opening. In (A), EGG waveform in the lower left, the frequency in the upper left, the amplitude in the upper right, and patient notes in the lower right are displayed on these images.

Recording of Images

Recorded images are generally used by clinicians or researchers who want to make visual perceptual observations that describe the gross features of the laryngeal movements.

Recording equipment should be chosen not only with consideration for the initial equipment cost outlay but also to the subsequent expenses of recording tapes and for storage of the recorded images. High-resolution recorders are now readily affordable. Super VHS and Super 8 recorders provide more lines of information, and therefore achieve better resolution, than the standard 1/2-inch VHS. The supers provide nearly identical resolution to the 3/4-inch VHS, and poorer resolution than the high-definition recorders. To get the best resolution, the Super VHS recorders must be used with Super VHS tapes; standard tapes reduce the resolution.

Several special features enhance clinical recording and analysis. Single-frame advance permits clinicians to view the images in slow motion: Freeze frame facilitates tracing of single images for comparing recordings made at different times and monitoring the effects of treatment. Fast-forward and reverse search features allow clinicians to rapidly access and review critical samples of interest. Character generators provide a good means of patient identification. Time-code generators allow clinicians to easily make measurements of timing features and to easily return to specific frames. Computerized video frame and character identification, such as Video Find®, facilitates instant retrieval of specific subjects recorded on different dates.

Video printers are no longer considered to be a luxury. Video printers permit clinicians to include stroboscopic data in flat graphic form in the patient's chart, provide reference for change in status of laryngeal disease, and facilitate communication among other health care workers. The most important factor is resolution: The better the resolution is, the better is the image and the ability to document small changes. Of nearly equal importance is the ability to record multiple images on the same print. This allows viewing of successive frames of a cycle of apparent motion as illustrated throughout this book. The following pages provide examples (Figures 3-9 to 3-24) obtained from video printers using various pathologies to illustrate technical problems one can encounter.

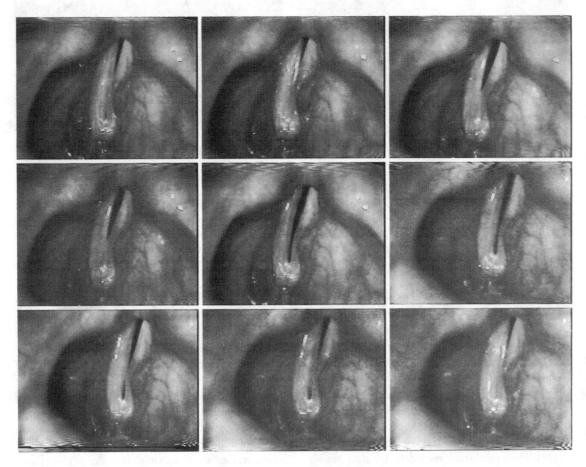

A

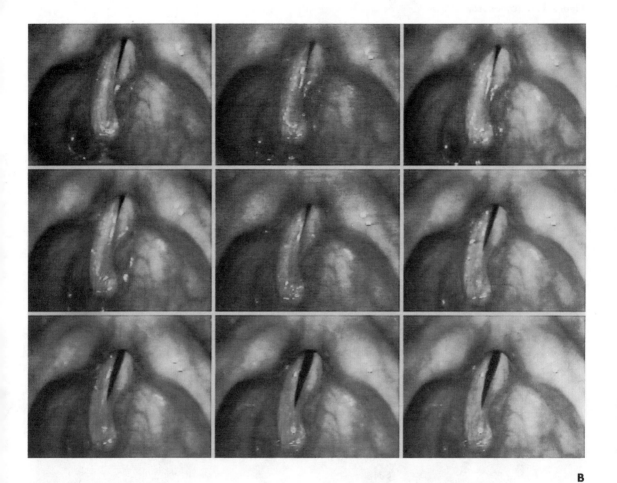

B

Figure 3–9. (A) A dark distant view of a case of a herniated ventricle could be mistakenly identified as a hypertrophied false vocal fold. Opening the lens provides a brighter picture (B). Using a magnifying lens enhances the clinical picture (C).

Figure 3–9. *(continued)*

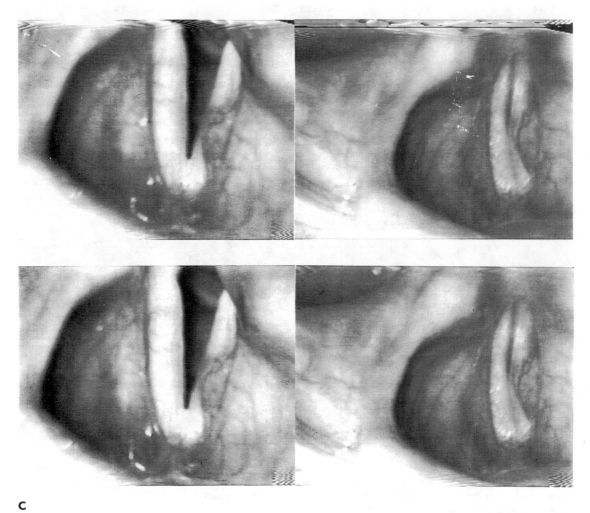

C

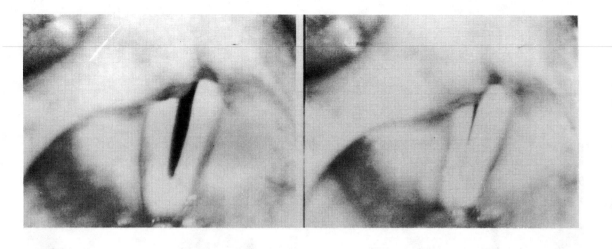

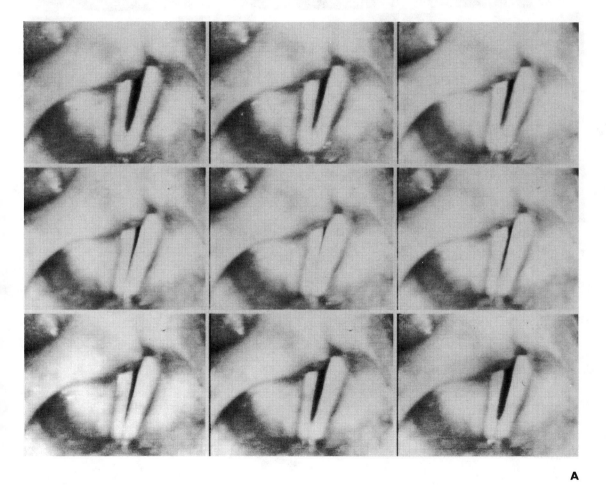

A

Figure 3–10. Video recordings demonstrate that the brightness level was too intense (A) and obscured some important detail on the vocal fold mucosa (B).

Figure 3–10. (continued)

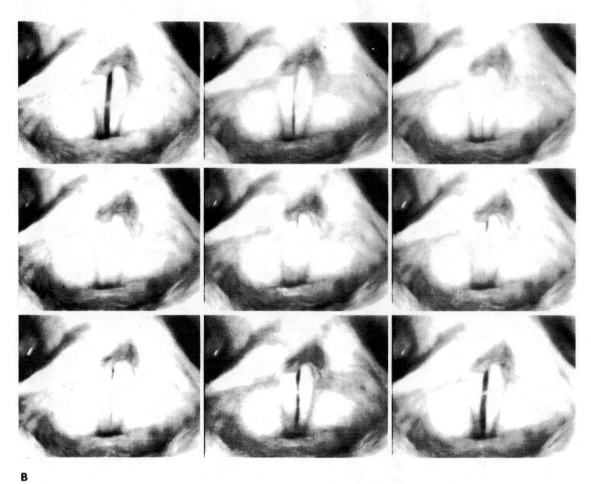

B

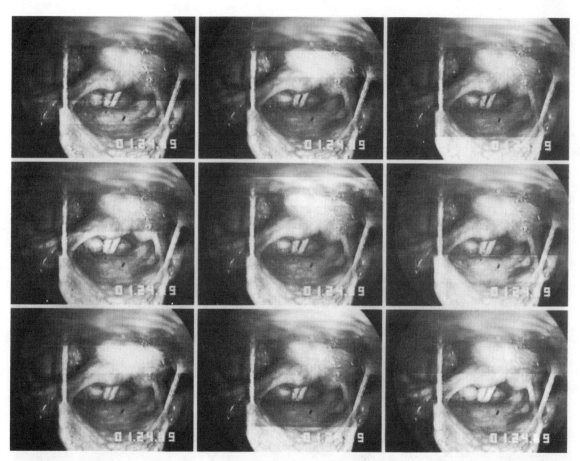

Figure 3–11. Small amplitude of movement is not easily visualized in this distant image of the vocal folds of a geriatric female. Using magnification or bringing the lens into closer approximation to the vocal folds would correct this problem.

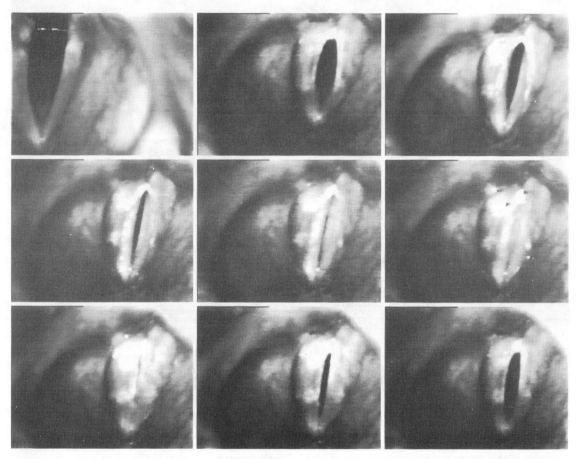

Figure 3–12. Movement patterns of the vocal folds of this male with chronic laryngitis cannot be easily visualized because the image is dark. This was produced with a stroboscopic bulb that was not producing maximum light.

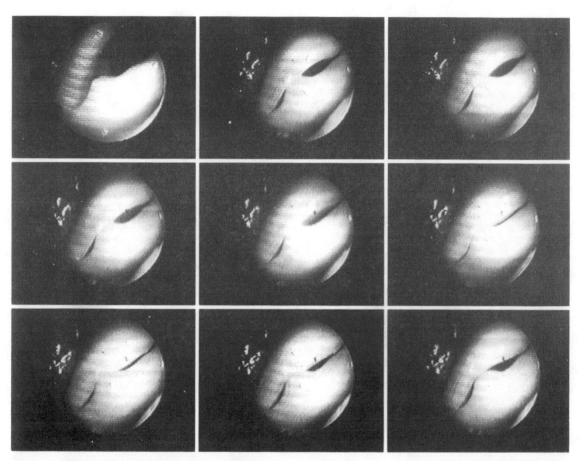

Figure 3–13. This recording was made with a flexible fiberscope closely approximating the lesion. Close approximation causes a visual distortion of the structure. This location may be necessary to differentiate cysts from nodules.

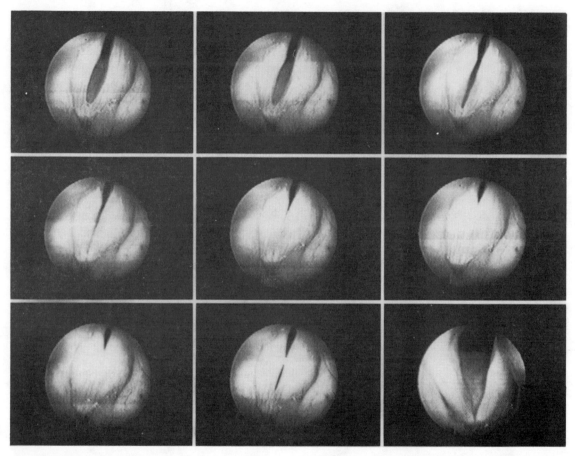

Figure 3–14. Illustration of good quality recording inadequately magnified. In a case of vocal fold edema and sulcus vocalis, increased magnification with a lower intensity of brightness would enhance the image and the clinician's ability to observe the effect of the two problems.

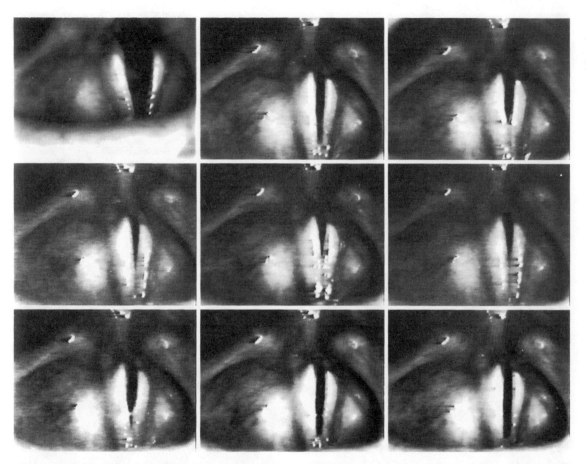

Figure 3–15. This video recording shows an image that is blurred from the developing process. Comparison of the printed image to the image on the monitor should lead the clinician to make a second print after making proper adjustments on the video printer.

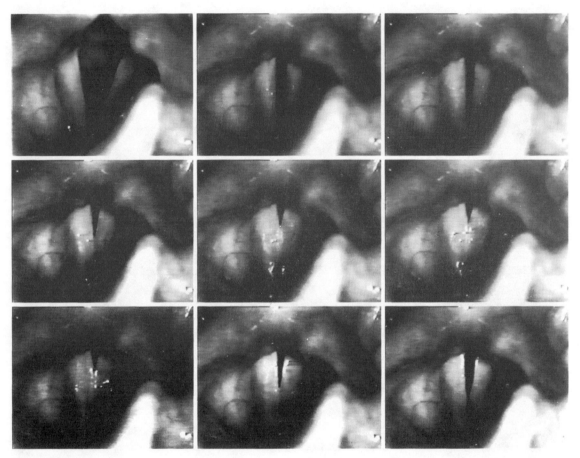

Figure 3-16. The rigid endoscope used in making this recording was placed at a slight angle. The angle, combined with an epiglottis that did not retract during /i/ production yielded a dark shadow with a distorted representation of the right vocal fold, which appears larger. Note that even with these technical problems, opening-closing patterns are apparent.

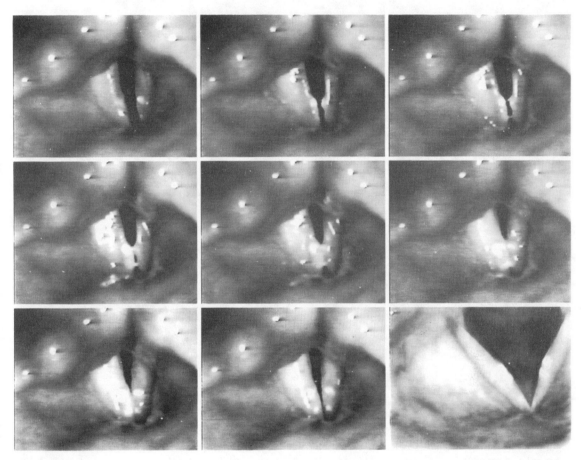

Figure 3-17. Image is not in optimal focus, making it difficult to differentiate mucus from thickenings of the mucosal membrane.

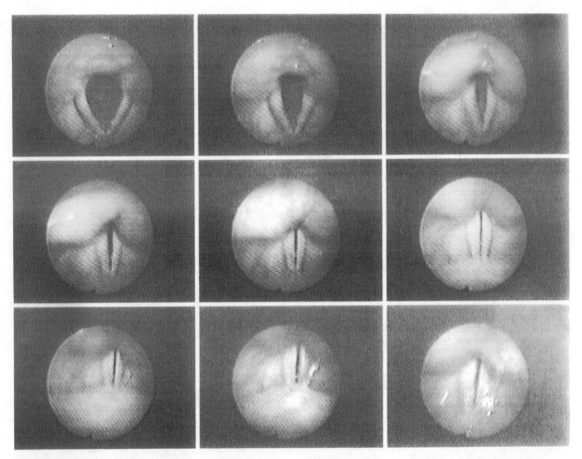

Figure 3–18. This flexible fiberscopic image could be enhanced with magnification. Clinicians would find it difficult to make meaningful observations of the vocal fold edge and mucosal wave as shown here. Amplitude of vibration, abduction and adduction, and opening-closing patterns could be discerned with magnification.

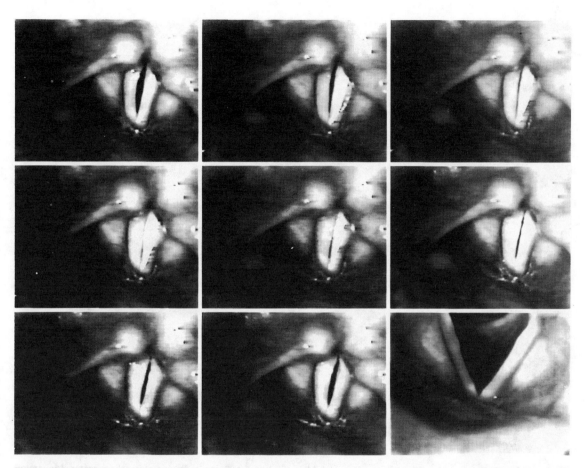

Figure 3–19. This case of vocal fold stiffness clearly demonstrates asymmetrical vibration. Amplitude of movement of the left vocal fold is not apparent. Mucus blurs the image. Having the patient clear his or her throat would improve visualization of the posterior half of the left vocal fold.

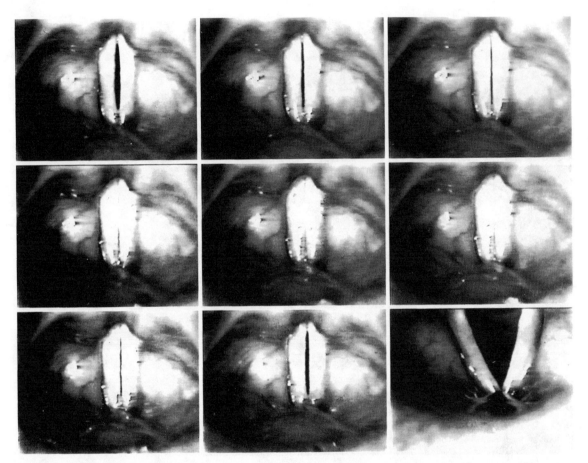

Figure 3-20. This is a good clear image of vocal fold opening and closing. Lighting and focus are adequate. Magnification is needed. Endoscope position should be altered to permit viewing of vocal processes. Movement in a superior and posterior direction should bring the posterior glottis in clear view.

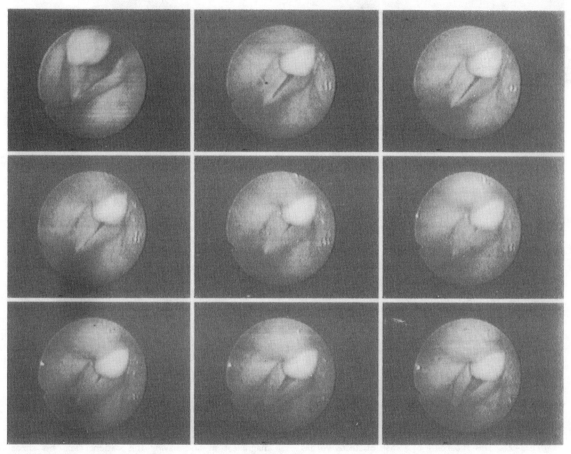

Figure 3–21. Although the image is not optimal it is adequate to view the effect that the contact granuloma has on inhibiting adduction.

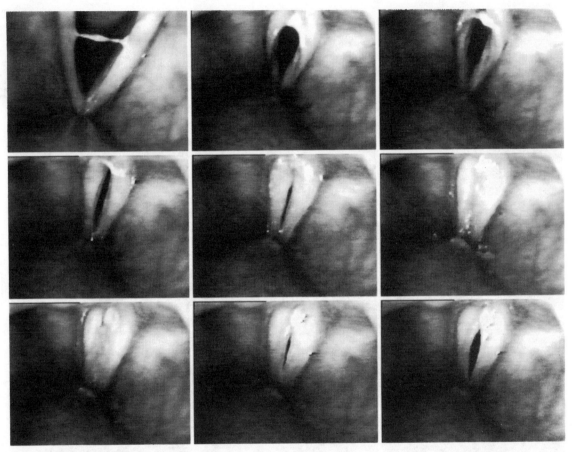

Figure 3–22. This recording of a case of sulcus vocalis demonstrates compensatory movement by the patient with what appears to be complete closure. Increased magnification and having this patient clear his throat revealed that the apparent closure was a mucous bridge obscuring the small opening.

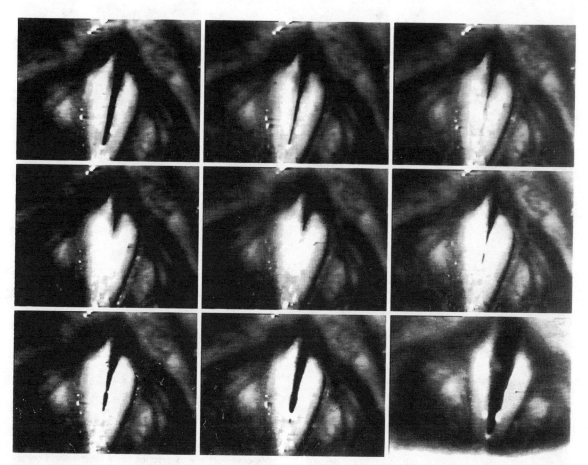

Figure 3–23. The darkness of this image was the result of two problems: tint level of the recorder and velar overhang preventing full illumination of the larynx. Repositioning the endoscope so that the velum is above the edge of the light and not at an angle would improve the image dramatically. It would provide the operator with visible detail and demonstrate symmetrical amplitude in contrast to the apparent asymmetry seen here.

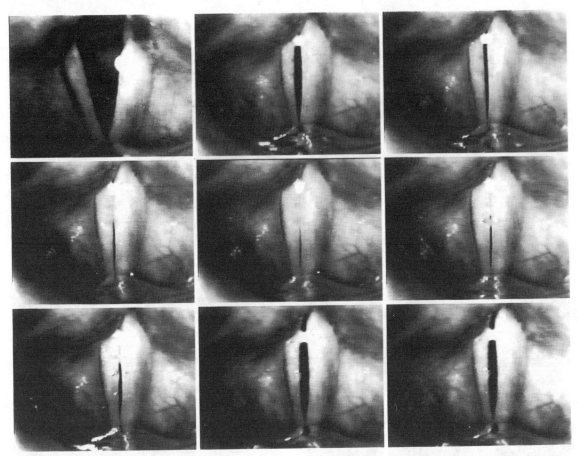

Figure 3–24. Posterior mucous stranding and incomplete glottal closure is seen in this video print despite endoscopic angle and low light level. Even when not of the best quality, videostroboscopy can provide valuable information. Obviously the better the image is, the better able observers are to describe vocal function and consequences of pathology.

Processing of Images

In the past 20 years, digital image processing has influenced many areas of medicine and speech pathology. Both the hardware and software for image processing are readily available for personal computers and are user-friendly. Radiographic images of the vocal tract have been processed digitally with resultant improvement in our ability to view movements of swallowing and to quantify changes in size, shape, or position of the tongue, lips, velum, and other parts of the body (Colton, Casper, Brewer, & Conture, 1989). Radiologists even use digital image processing to have X rays transmitted to them via telephone lines.

In theory, these image-processing techniques could easily be applied to the larynx to help quantify structure and movement and to communicate findings to other professionals. In practice, it is not so simple, because the vertical excursions of the larynx make absolute measurements difficult. Moreover, at present, the image enhancement programs are time-consuming and require a skilled technician to set the cursors to make the measurements (see Figure 3–25). Nevertheless, initial studies are encouraging (Casper, Brewer, & Colton, 1987; Conture, Schwartz, & Brewer, 1986; Rammage, Peppard, & Bless, 1992) and suggest that image processing — though time-consuming — might be useful for collecting and analyzing laryngeal images. Image processing can be used to determine opening-closing patterns, to identify the shape of glottal opening, to describe the glottal gap ratio, to estimate the areas of feature in the image, and, in some instances, to improve the visual quality. The limitations are not unlike those described by Booth and Childers (1979) in their classic article on automated analysis of ultra-high-speed laryngeal films. Handicaps include poor contrast caused by insufficient lighting during recording, multiple glottal openings, incomplete image of the glottis, mucus bridging of the vocal folds separating the glottis into several distinct openings, and nonuniform open and closing patterns.

Of particular interest is a software program called *Image®*. *Image®* is a public domain program for the Apple Macintosh® computer for acquiring, enhancing, analyzing, editing, and color coding of gray-scale images; performing standard image analyses; and doing histograms, contrast enhancement, density profiling, and digital filtering. It is available at no cost from Wayne Rasband[1] of the National Institutes of Health, Bethesda, MD. Like video technology, both hardware and software development change too rapidly to be described in a book.

SAFETY AND RISK MANAGEMENT

The safety and risk management factors in stroboscopic examination of the larynx must take into account both the people and the equipment. Special precautions are necessary for speech and language pathologists. Before undertaking these procedures, every practitioner must heed the precautions identified by the ASHA Ad Hoc Committee on Advances in Clinical Practice (1992a, b).

1. Inform institutional and/or regulatory bodies, such as state licensure boards, about these procedures as within the scope of practice;
2. Check with state licensure board(s) (where appropriate) to determine whether or not there are limitations on the scope of speech-language pathology practice that restrict the performance of these procedures;
3. Check professional liability insurance to ensure that there is no exclusion applicable to these procedures;
4. Follow the *Universal Precautions* to prevent the risk of disease transmission from blood/air-borne pathogens, contained in the Centers for Disease Control Morbidity and Mortality Weekly Report (1988) or ASHA's AIDS/HIV Update (1990);
5. Have immediate emergency medical assistance available;
6. Hold a current Basic Life Support Certificate; and
7. Obtain informed consent of the patient and maintain complete and appropriate documentation.

Regardless of the clinician's training within his or her discipline, before the equipment is used it should be checked by a qualified electronics engineer or clinic safety staff to ensure that the room and equipment are properly grounded and pose no personal safety threat.

Any part of the examination system that the patient will come into contact with should be thoroughly disinfected between patients. The wearing of gloves is recommended at all times. Hospitals generally provide rules and guidelines that should be followed, unless the examiner feels the requirements are not sufficiently stringent. Most endoscopes come with instructions for use of disinfectants with needed immersion times; these guides also should be followed carefully, for failure to do so may cause degradation of the fiberoptic bundles. For example, one manufacturer suggests the use of 70% alcohol, 0.5% chlorhexine in 60% alcohol, 3% Korsolin® or Cidex®, maximum 1 hour; users are cautioned that use of any other solution is at the user's own risk. Thus, the clinician has the difficult responsibility of

[1] Wayne Rasband, National Institutes of Health, Building 36, Room 2A03, 9000 Rockville Pike, Bethesda, MD 20892.

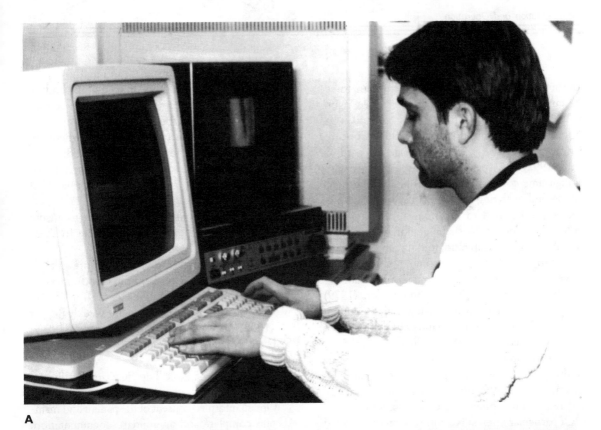

A

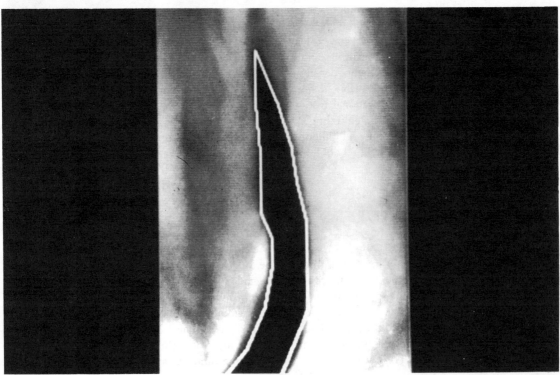

B

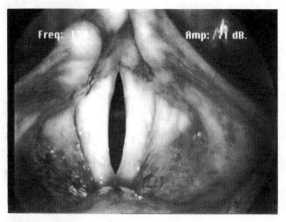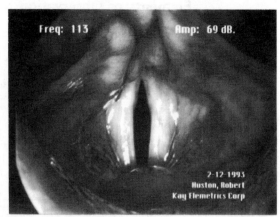

C

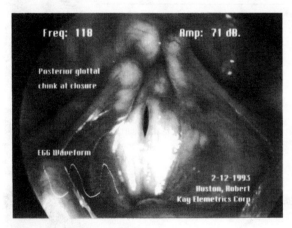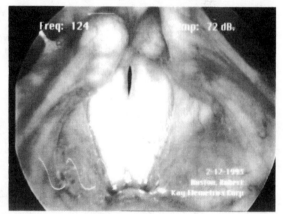

D

Figure 3–25. Technician operating an image processing program on a VAX Computer (A). Close-up of screen indicates edge detected to obtain area measurements (B). In (C), images where edge detection could be easily applied to define the entire glottis (left) and 7/8 of the glottis (right). (D) Images where edge detection would be possible for the posterior gap but difficult anteriorly because of the brightness of the image.

selecting a disinfectant that will protect the patient, comply with local regulations, and not be harmful to the instrumentation.

In dealing with issues concerning hygiene safety, perhaps the most important concept to impress on clinicians is that there is no time at which the risk is not present. One cannot presume that disinfectant measures should be enlisted *only* when a patient has been positively identified as carrying a virus or bacterium — rather that these measures should be rigorously followed as routine laboratory practice.

When the clinician and staff are comfortable with all preparation of instrumentation and planned operation of videostroboscopy, then clinical procedures can begin.

APPENDIX 3–1

Elements of Observation for Rating Scales

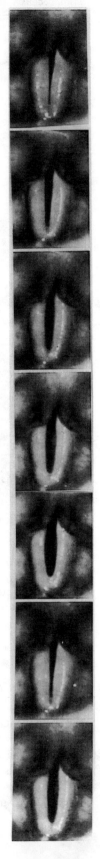

NAME
DOB **HOSPITAL ID**

	(0)	(1)	(2)	(3)	(4)	(5)
CLOSURE LEVEL	Glottic Plane					Off Plane

	(0)	(1)	(2)	(3)	(4)	(5)
VOCAL FOLD EDGE	Smooth Straight					Rough Irregular

	(0)	(1)	(2)	(3)	(4)	(5)
SUPRAGLOTTIC INVOLVEMENT	None					Dysphonia Plicae Ventricularis

		(0)	(1)	(2)	(3)	(4)	(5)
	LEFT	(0)	(1)	(2)	(3)	(4)	(5)
AMPLITUDE		Normal	Slightly Decreased	Moderately Decreased	Severely Decreased	Barely Perceptible	No Visible Movement
	RIGHT	(0)	(1)	(2)	(3)	(4)	(5)

		(0)	(1)	(2)	(3)	(4)	(5)
	LEFT	(0)	(1)	(2)	(3)	(4)	(5)
MUCOSAL WAVE		Normal	Slightly Decreased	Moderately Decreased	Severely Decreased	Barely Perceptible	Absent
	RIGHT	(0)	(1)	(2)	(3)	(4)	(5)

		(0)	(1)	(2)	(3)	(4)	(5)
	LEFT	(0)	(1)	(2)	(3)	(4)	(5)
NON-VIBRATING PORTION		None	20%	40%	60%	80%	100%
	RIGHT	(0)	(1)	(2)	(3)	(4)	(5)

	(−5)	(−4)	(−3)	(−2)	(−1)	(0)	(1)	(2)	(3)	(4)	(5)
CLOSURE PHASE	Open Phase Predominates (Whisper dysphonia)					**Normal**				Closed Phase Predominates (Glottal fry-extreme hyper adduction)	

NARRATIVE REPORT

STUDY QUESTIONS

1. Through the use of stroboscopy in the clinical setting one can:

   a. Observe hyperfunction of the larynx.

   b. Recognize changes in stiffness.

   c. Identify pathologies.

   d. Observe the vibratory patterns of the vocal folds.

   e. All of the above.

2. The basic equipment of a stroboscope consists of a light source, an electronic control unit, a foot pedal, and a(n):

   a. Anesthetic.

   b. Monitor.

   c. Microphone.

   d. Camera.

3. The stroboscope view of the larynx can be recorded from:

   a. A laryngeal mirror.

   b. A rigid or flexible endoscope.

   c. An operating microscope.

   d. All of the above.

4. A setting that must be checked to ensure maximum performance of the stroboscope is the:

   a. Phase.

   b. Chair position.

   c. Light source frequency.

   d. Tongue position.

5. During voice production, as vocal pitch increases:

   a. Vocal fold length decreases.

   b. Mucosal wave is reduced.

   c. Glottal closure remains constant.

   d. None of the above.

6. Mucosal wave is reduced or absent with the pathology(ies) of:

   a. Vocal fold edema.

   b. Hyperfunction.

   c. Carcinoma.

   d. Anxiety about the examination.

   e. All of the above.

7. When making judgments on a laryngeal image and asymmetry is observed, one should:

   a. Suspect a pathology.

   b. Consider the larynx to be normal if it is without other observed variation.

   c. Refer the patient to an otolaryngologist.

   d. Set up a series of muscle-strengthening exercises to do in therapy.

8. Glottal chinks are commonly seen in (choose all that apply):

   a. Geriatic males.

   b. Children.

   c. Females.

   d. None of the above.

9. Stroboscopy can help show efficacy of treatment when:

   a. Comparing pre- and post-treatment samples.

   b. Using a rating scale on many different vocal parameters.

   c. Using a standard protocol including changes in pitch and loudness.

   d. All of the above.

10. Which of the following is a patient factor that does not affect videostroboscopic procedures?

    a. Fear of the procedure.

    b. Hyperactive gag reflex.

    c. Gender.

11. Optical distortion and apparent motion are artifacts that can often occur because of:

    a. Placement of the endoscope.

    b. An omega-shaped epiglottis.

    c. A small oral cavity.

    d. The choice of camera lens.

12. Which of the following is not a precaution for performing stroboscopic examinations of the larynx?

    a. Check with state licensure boards to determine limitations on the scope of practice.

    b. Check professional liability insurance to ensure coverage.

    c. Enroll in a training seminar on the use of stroboscopy in clinical practice.

    d. Obtain written patient consent prior to examination.

Clinical Procedures for Observation and Administration

The clinical procedures for the videostroboscopic examination involves an understanding of what is to be observed, what protocol is appropriate to given symptoms and to a patient's individual needs, and what administrative elements are necessary to incorporate videostroboscopy into a clinical setting.

OBSERVATION

Quasiobjective records on the nature of laryngeal disease have great importance in group discussion, demonstrations, and follow-up studies of the problem. For both accurate assessment of voice disorders and appropriate administration of medical care, observation and recording by videostroboscopy must meet certain basic standards.

General Requirements

The method of examining and obtaining recordings on the larynx should meet the following requirements (Saito, Fukuda, Kitahara, & Isogai, 1984):

1. The examination should be performed with the patient in as natural a posture as possible and without causing the individual any discomfort.
2. The field of vision should not be obscured by the epiglottis.
3. The handling procedures should be simple.
4. Clear, magnified images should be obtained for examination and recording.
5. The laryngeal view should include the arytenoids, the anterior commissure, and the maximal glottal width (Figure 4-1).

Precise photographic documentation of the larynx and adjacent structures enhances diagnosis and management of laryngeal disorders. Its value in permanent record keeping, teaching, and research is well-known. Laryngeal photography includes microscopic photography, telescopic photography, and fiberscopic photography (Andrews & Gould, 1977; Davidson, Bone, & Nahum, 1974; Dellon, Clifford, Chretien, 1975; Gould, Kojima, & Lambiase, 1979; Konrad, Hople, & Bussen, 1981; Saito, Isogai, &

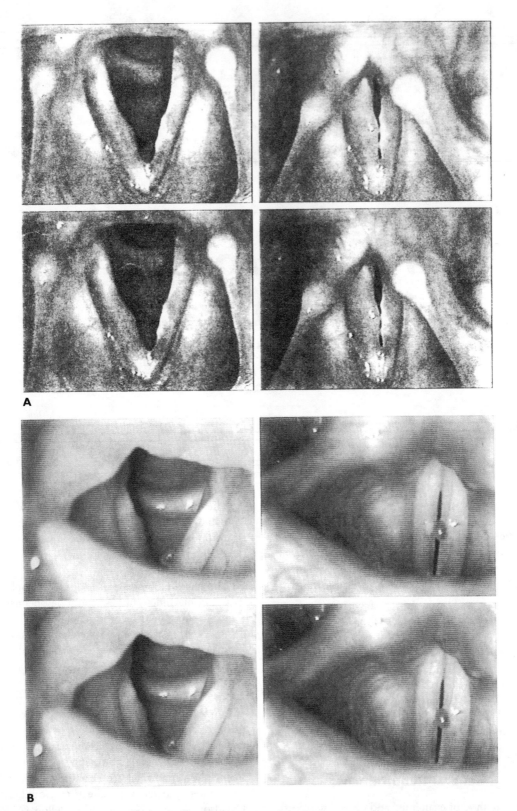

Figure 4-1. Videoprints of the larynx illustrate the ideal image with clear view of the entire length of the vocal folds: (A) image positioned in the center of the screen, (B) compromised image in which the anterior commissure is not visible because of the epiglottis, and (C) off-center view taken at an angle.

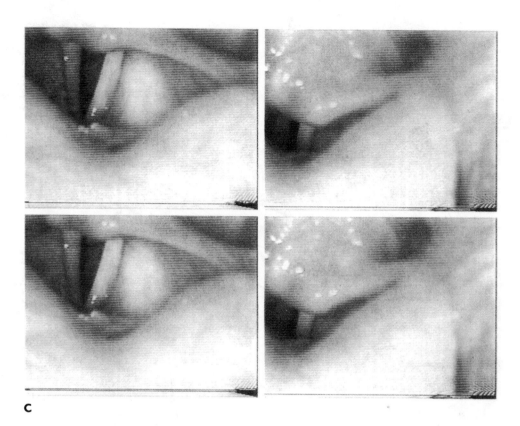

C

Fukuda, 1981; Sawashima, Totsuka, Kobayoshi, & Hirose, 1968; Silberman, Wilf, & Tucker, 1967; Tobin, 1980; White & Knight, 1984; Williams, Farquharson, & Anthony, 1975; Yanagisawa, Owens, Strothers, & Honda, 1983). These photographic procedures can be used in an office setting and can be combined with videostroboscopic recording equipment to produce images of movement. Furthermore, the videostroboscopic recording equipment can be combined with EGG to account for cycle-to-cycle variations in vibration.

Telescopic Recording

Two procedures are typically used in telescopic recordings with the straight, rigid endoscope: examiner-conducted and self-directed. The choice depends on the purpose of the testing, the equipment available, the examiner, and the patient.

Examiner-Conducted Evaluation

For the examiner-conducted evaluation, the patient is seated upright in front of the examiner with the neck slightly extended and head tilted slightly back (Figure 4–2). A microphone is placed on the patient's neck just inferior to the thyroid cartilage. The patient is asked to sustain /i/ while the examiner checks the digital frequency reading to ensure that microphone placement is appropriate. If the placement is appropriate the microphone is secured by Velcro® strap, surgical adhesive, or electromyograph (EMG) electrode stickers. It is also possible to ask the patient to hold the microphone, but this practice is generally not advised because the patient might be unable to maintain correct placement, necessitating additional and repetitive testing. The patient-held microphone might also cause artificial

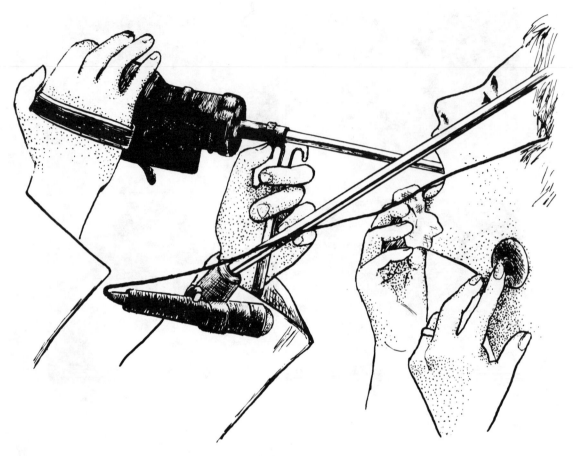

Figure 4–2. In the examiner-conducted evaluation using a rigid endoscope, the tongue and the microphone are self-held by the patient.

asymmetries because of the unilateral elevated arm and shoulder position.

When the microphone is in place, the examination begins. The patient extends the tongue and the examiner or patient grasps it with a 4 × 4 gauze pad. While the subject breathes quietly, the scope is inserted with the lens side up. As the endoscope is being inserted into the oral cavity, the examiner gently rotates the scope until the lens is facing the larynx, taking care not to scrape the dorsum of the tongue. Inserting the lens side up reduces the probability of any mucous collecting on the tip of the scope. The clinician uses the epiglottis as a landmark to signify that the scope is close to the correct position. The position will vary with the type of scope used. Figure 4–3 shows how the larynx is imaged with the 90° scope parallel to the surface of the superior aspect of the vocal folds, placed at the juncture of the hard

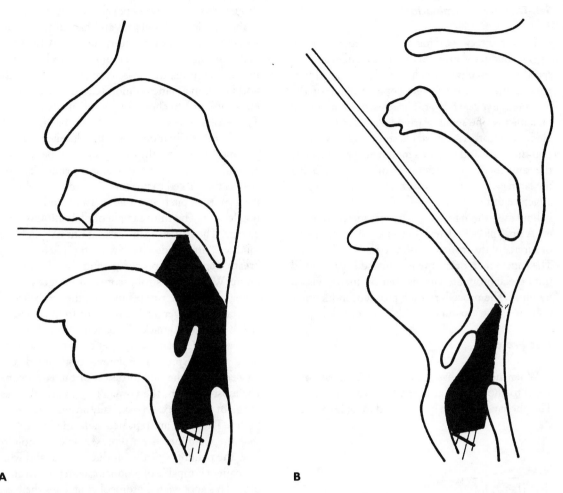

Figure 4–3. Two rigid endoscope placements maximize their respective angle of views of the larynx: (A) 90°, and (B) 70° endoscope.

and soft palate, and the 70° scope is placed at a greater angle and approximates the posterior pharyngeal wall.

The foot pedal is depressed to activate the observation light. The patient is asked to phonate /i/ to initiate the stroboscopic light, and to permit recording of vocal fold vibration. No topical anesthesia is necessary for about 80% of typical adults. When necessary, surface anesthesia with 4% Lidocaine® spray is sufficient to suppress the gag reflex. In some individuals, the anesthesia causes the patient to produce excess secretions, making examination of the vocal

folds difficult. However, for most patients, topical anesthesia makes the examination easier and the vocal folds easier to view, and does not have an observable effect on vocal fold vibration.

To prevent fogging of the lens, several options might be necessary: air insufflation, heated dental beads, a solid antifogging agent, heating the telescope by placing it for 30 sec against the buccal tissue, dipping it in warm water, or blowing hot air across the lens tip. The air insufflation is not advised for patients who have easily elicited gag response, as the air impinging on the pharyngeal wall can exacerbate the reflex.

Self-Directed Examination

The self-directed examination procedure (Figure 4–4) is conducted in much the same manner as high-speed photography of the larynx. The major difference is the use of the telescope in place of the mounted laryngeal mirror. The telescope is mounted on a microscope stand or tripod placed in front of a video monitor. An adjustable stool is used to position the scope and patient's mouth at approximately the same level. The patient sits on the stool facing the laryngoscope and monitor. The patient is shown a picture of the desired view. The examiner stands behind the patient to assist in placement when needed. A small piece of dental wax is placed on the inferior surface of the frontal incisors to protect the teeth. The patient then opens the mouth and leans forward until the appropriate view is seen on the television monitor. The procedure then proceeds in identical fashion to the examiner-conducted method.

Test Protocol

When the larynx has been visualized, the patient is asked to phonate /i/ at normal pitch and loudness. The phonation should be sustained for at least 2 sec,

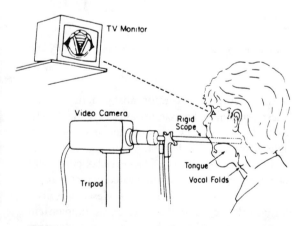

Figure 4–4. Patient-conducted evaluation using a rigid endoscope. This visual feedback system was used by Bastian (1987a) for modifying vocal behavior. The monitor is placed where clinician and patient both have a full view of the larynx.

though this is not always possible for dysphonic patients with large glottal gaps and high airflow or for speakers with weak respiratory support. After a normal recording is made, the examiner checks for aperiodicity by using the phase control to visualize the vocal folds in a static position (e.g., the beat is turned on and off) to check for periodicity of vibration. This is followed by moving slowly through the different phases of vibration, especially closely inspecting the open phase. It is the open phase that permits the examiner to observe the infraglottic margin. The patient is then asked to produce the same vowel starting at normal pitch and loudness and gradually getting louder. The third sample of phonation is pitch change. The patient again starts at normal pitch and loudness, and gradually elevates the pitch, takes a breath, repeats the procedure and then lowers the pitch. With some stroboscopes, it is necessary to change the mode of operation of the stroboscopic generator to cover a large range of frequencies. To check for glottal attack, the patient is asked to produce a syllable chain of /i/ repetitions produced at a rapid rate. The protocol is limited to sustained vowels because of the oral intrusion of the endoscope. For most speakers, the vowel /i/ provides the best image of the larynx. Occasionally an /ai/ or /uo/ is better. The tasks are repeated as needed to ensure that the examiner has a representative sample of how the patient typically produces voice and what the patient is capable of producing with present anatomy. This abbreviated protocol completes the basic screening tasks; for some patients, extended observation of laryngeal dynamics is needed. The protocol is designed to maximize differences that might be unique to particular pathologies as is discussed later in this chapter.

Injury to teeth is a potential complication of stroboscopic examination with a rigid endoscope. This is a common complication of endotracheal intubation. Several methods have been devised to prevent such injury, including use of rubber or plastic guards (Evers, Racz, Glazer, & Dobkin, 1967), tape (Jephcott, 1984), and dental wax. The technique most applicable to videostroboscopy is the use of dental wax. A piece of heat-sensitive dental wax is softened with warm water and is then pressed gently against the frontal incisors. The examination then proceeds as usual.

As an alternative, the examiner can grasp the tongue between the middle finger and thumb and place the index finger between the frontal incisors and the endoscope. This also helps in stabilization of the endoscope.

Fiberscopic Recording

The flexible laryngoscope is useful for making videolaryngoscopic recordings and is easily mastered. The advantages relative to the rigid endoscope are that the endoscope can be placed closer to the vocal fold and the speech structures don't have any restrictions (Figure 4–5), making it possible to visualize the larynx during connected speech and whistling tasks. Major limitations cited by Cantarella (1987) and echoed by others are: lack of image definition, low color fidelity, wide-angle distortion, inaccurate assessment of small le-

sions, slight color changes of fold are difficult to detect, and structures of the hemilarynx close to the endoscope tip appear more bulky. These problems are not insurmountable.

The fiberscope, which appears nearly ideal in concept, requires more than just basic mannequin practice to appreciate the altered view of the upper airway structures. Although it can be used orally, the nasal route is preferred to avoid injury to the fiberoptic bundles, and to leave the speech structures unencumbered.

Fiberscopic recordings are conducted by both speech pathologists and laryngologists, though there are some clear differences in protocol. Most speech pathologists use fiberscopes to observe patterns of velopharyngeal closure, swallowing, or phonation, as well as to conduct visual feedback therapy. These extended observations are time consuming and most clinicians allot an hour or more time to

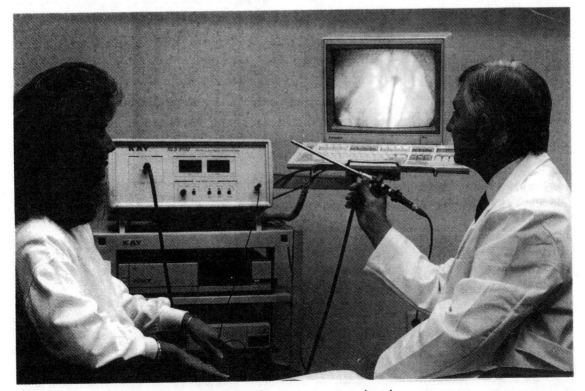

Figure 4–5. The flexible fiberscope leaves speech apparatus unencumbered.

execute the procedure. Because they are not physicians, they cannot use topical anesthesia except under a physician's supervision. Thus, the procedures evolving from this specialty generally require a lengthier examination and do not employ topical spray.

By contrast, physicians use the fiberscope to make a medical diagnosis, generally use topical anesthetics, and schedule considerably less time for the examination procedure. In some cases, the procedure is done by a team. The otolaryngologist anesthetizes the patient and inserts the fiberscope, and the speech pathologist devises the test protocol and attempts to use behavioral management techniques and to apply manual compression tests while the larynx is being visualized.

The patient is seated comfortably in a conventional examining chair, and the procedure is explained to him or her. The tip of the laryngoscope is lubricated to facilitate its passage. The nasal cavities are sometimes sprayed with vasoconstrictor prior to inspection of the nasal cavity, permitting the examiner to see any septal spur or deviation and identify the less obstructed side for passage of the fiberscope. One method of administering topical anesthetic is to spray 2% tetracaine HCl (Pontocaine®) onto the nasal mucosa, allowing some of it to trickle into the nasopharynx and hypopharynx. Tetracaine is applied again and allowed to flow into the hypopharynx. Another method is to place pledgets containing 4% Lidocaine® in the nose for 5 minutes. An alternative local anesthesia for the nose is 5% cocaine. In instances when clinicians wish to closely inspect the vocal folds, and anticipate touching the vocal fold surface, a transtracheal injection of 2% or 4% Lidocaine® is placed through the cricothyroid membrane, unless contraindicated by a local disease or traumatic processes (Raj, Forestner, Watson, Morris, & Jenkins, 1974). To reduce gagging, the patient gargles with 10 ml of 4% Lidocaine® for 1 minute; this is repeated once. If the patient is unable to gargle, the palate and oropharynx are swabbed or sprayed with the solution. Occasionally, anxious patients even require sedation by diazepam or a narcotic.

The examiner stands in front of or slightly to the side of the seated patient with the camera cradled under the arm or supported on the shoulder; the fiberscope bundle can then be easily manipulated and steadied with the clinician's left hand, and the right hand can rotate the tip deflector (White & Knight, 1984). In this way the scope can be passed to the nasopharynx, the tip deflected inferiorly, and then advanced to a level where the epiglottis can be visualized. The scope is then further advanced and positioned until the desired view of the larynx is obtained. When the vocal folds are visualized, the test protocol is initiated. Usually, up to this point, the recorder has been in the "pause" phase, so no recording tape is running. The recorder is then switched to "record" until the examination is complete. The larynx is video- and audiotaped during: (1) identification of name and date; (2) respiration, both resting and forced; (3) counting 1 to 10; (4) prolongation of /i/ at habitual and maximum pitch and loudness levels; (5) production of glottal coup; (6) coughing; (7) reading sentences; (8) singing the first phrase of "Happy Birthday"; (9) laryngeal diadochokinesis; and (10) whistling.

If stroboscopic images are poor because of insufficient light sensitivity in the system, the distal end of the endoscope is adjusted until it nearly approximates the vocal folds. Close approximation of the vocal folds enhances the image, but also increases distortion and the possibility of eliciting a laryngospasm. The examiner can also compensate for inadequate illumination by using the zoom capability of the focus mechanism to decrease the image diameter or by using a different lens to increase brightness.

One of the greatest values of stroboscopy is the ability to make comparisons of the structure pre- and posttreatment. To make valid comparisons it is essential that clinicians use the same protocol — maintaining similar pitch and loudness levels — during all test sessions. (See Chapter 3 for additional issues pertaining to reliability of recordings.)

PROTOCOL

The precise protocol selected will depend on the patient and the pathology. For example, in cases of paralysis, it is important to carefully check how pitch is changed and phonation is initiated; whereas, in cases of spastic dysphonia, connected speech samples provide the most valuable information, and in cases of papilloma or scar tissue, close up views of aerodynamic segments during sustained vowels are most valuable. The clinician must be aware of the possibility of initiating laryngospasm. Developing the patients' ability to modify laryngeal movements with visual feedback also requires a specific protocol. Thus, protocol must be adapted individually for each patient.

Considerations

Questions to be answered in the stroboscopic examination naturally evolve from the learned clinician. The clinician who is knowledgeable about the anatomy and physiology of the larynx, pathophysiology of laryngeal diseases, and assessment instruments will use the stroboscope to help define the issues. For example, questions posed in cases of suspected laryngeal paralysis might include: What happens when the patient attempts to increase pitch? Is the mucosal wave reduced? Does the patient provide evidence of increased medial compression without hyperfunction when attempting to increase loudness? Can arytenoid dislocation or fixation be ruled out? Is the vibratory movement asymmetrical? Questions posed for a person with nodules might include: Do the lesions appear soft and pliable? Does the closed phase appear long and abusive? Does vocal initiation appear to be hyperfunctional and mechanically traumatic to the vocal fold tissue? Is the amplitude greatly indicting overdrive? Can vocal fold cysts be ruled out? Is there any evidence of stiffness along the vibrating surface of the vocal folds? Thus, pathology dictates the protocol, and the clinician must understand how the pathology affects the body/cover relationships to develop the best protocol and to interpret the resultant images.

Laryngospasms

Laryngospasms are an inherent danger in conducting endoscopic examination. There are no known incidence figures of the number encountered relative to the number of patients examined. Predisposing factors seem to be the presence of mucus and saliva, which might physically stimulate the larynx and cause laryngospasm and laryngeal dyskinesias.

Other factors, such as the irritability of the inhalation agents themselves, the depth of anesthesia, and mechanical trauma (e.g., tip of the endoscope touching the mucosa), appear to also play a role. Suzuki, Saito, Hayasaki, and Murakami (1964) write about the reflex arc of laryngospasm, indicating that it is almost certainly mediated by the afferent superior laryngeal nerve. The researchers separate laryngospasm from routine reflex glottic closure by the intensity of stimulation and the maintenance of a persistent response.

With the use of microscopic suspension surgery for laryngeal lesions, Colman and Reynolds (1985) notice an unacceptably high incidence of laryngospasms. They postulate that the high level was caused by the larynx being manipulated directly and the fresh surgical wounds providing enough superior laryngeal nerve stimulation to trigger this dangerous reflex. To counteract this problem, they began to topically apply a small amount of cocaine solution (10% in adults, 4% in children) to the vocal folds, arytenoids, and false fold. This reduced the problem. The cocaine was either dripped on the endolaryngeal surfaces or applied on a cotton pledget wiped across the mucosal surfaces of the endolarynx. Colman and Reynolds (1985) observe no side effects from use of topical cocaine on the mucosal surfaces of the larynx. They also note no unexpected arrhythmias or no incidence of cardiac depressions or seizures, though note that all are possible. They conclude that the small narcotic amount absorbed from the laryngeal mucosa is minimal in terms of total systemic dosage.

Visual Feedback

Videostroboscopic recordings are not only useful in assessment; they are equally valuable as treatment tools in modifying movement patterns. Visual feedback is particularly useful with cases of hyperfunction and laryngeal dyskinesias. Most important in the physical arrangement is positioning the video monitor where both the clinician and patient have the larynx in full view (see Figure 4–5). When the larynx is visualized, the treatment procedure can begin. First, the structures of interest are identified for the patient. The explanations should be simple and structures identified kept to a minimum. The patient is instructed about which behaviors are to be modified and asked to replace accustomed performance with the target behavior. For example, a patient exhibiting a long closed phase thought to be causing mechanical trauma might be asked to initiate a soft phonation with an /h/while visually monitoring the decreased closed period. Patients with paradoxical vocal fold motion need to recognize they can learn to control the glottal opening. Contrasting glottal chinks with phonation while visually monitoring the images is beneficial to these patients. When the clinician believes the patient understands the target, he or she is asked to glide from one behavior to the other. Clinicians using this treatment have found that it facilitates rapid acquisition of a desired behavior, it motivates the patients, and it helps increase their knowledge about the larynx. Clinicians using this technique stress the importance of fading the feedback as quickly as possible to prevent the patient from becoming dependent on the visual image and to foster development of dependence on the kinesthetic and proprioceptive feedback accompanying the target gesture.

INTERPRETATION OF DATA

Interpretation of data takes more skill than any of the other procedures (Figure 4-6). It necessitates integrating knowledge of disease, anatomy, physiology, phonation, and other issues that impact the functional use of the system. One cannot hope to make valid and reliable interpretation without considerable practice. With 20 hours of viewing training, most observers can reach 90% agreement or higher on symmetry, closure phase, amplitude of vibration, mucosal wave, and closure pattern. Plane level of approximation takes additional training. To reach these levels, it is necessary to view a variety of stroboscopic recordings that demonstrate the range of motion seen for normal speakers at different ages for both males and females and also for different pathological conditions causing changes to the body and cover.

ADMINISTRATION

The reality of medical examination in our world is that keeping track of time, keeping records, and charg-

ing fees are necessary. We would be remiss in presenting a text on videostroboscopic assessment for the clinician if we did not address the realities of the procedure's administration.

Time

The time allotted for videostroboscopic examination must be long enough to acquire accurate and appropriate records of the patient's voice and larynx, but short enough to control costs and inconvenience.

The time needed to complete the protocol depends on a number of factors: the patient's anatomy, the patient's ability to follow instructions, the examiner's skill, the protocol dictated by the pathology, and the need to attempt trial behavioral management or manual compression tests. For a brief assessment procedure of sustained vowels, the entire recording procedure can be completed in 10–15 minutes. For other subjects who require trial therapy or prolonged observation of laryngeal dynamics, the procedure may be more lengthy, perhaps 30–45 minutes.

When the recording is complete, the records must be examined and rated and the observations entered into the patient's record. The rating procedures, parameters, and forms are discussed elsewhere in this text. It generally takes about 10 minutes to complete this part of the procedure.

Record Keeping

At least three types of patient record keeping are advisable: a short checklist (Figure 4-7), a narrative paragraph (Figure 4-8), and a video print (Figure 4-9). R. E. Stone at Vanderbilt University has developed a computer data base record for this purpose (see Appendix 4-1). These reports need not be mutually exclusive and can be combined to provide the maximum information for future comparison and to facilitate communication with other healthcare providers. The short checklist has the advantage of taking little additional time; it is a useful means of keeping a "second set" of records for communication with someone who is familiar with interpretation of stroboscopic findings. The more elaborate version of the narrative is necessary for those who do not use the stroboscope regularly and need assistance with interpretation.

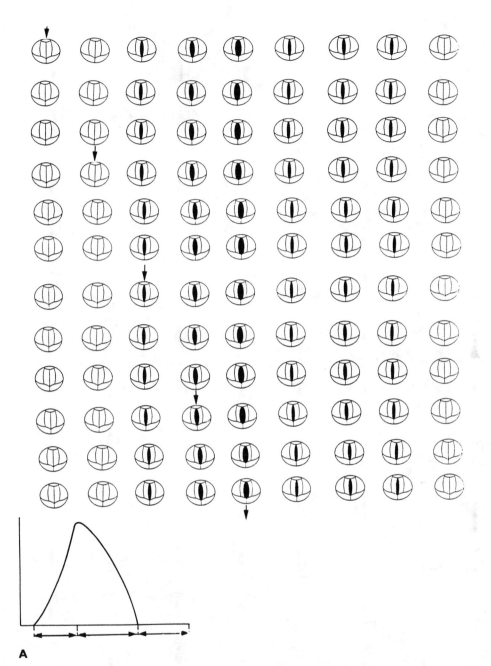

A

Figure 4–6. Examples of different movement patterns. In these figures (A–D) each row depicts image fragments from one glottal cycle of a male speaker at 100 Hz. The graph at the bottom depicts the derived glottal cycle. In high-speed photography each row would consist of 20 frames taken at a speed of 2,000 frames per second. Standard videostroboscopy at 33 frames per second would sample one frame from every four cycles (in the schematic, from every four rows). In perfectly regular voice, (A) videostroboscopic sampling (vertical arrows) would yield uniform patterns of observation. In typical, slightly irregu-lar voice, (B) videostroboscopic sampling could miss cycle-to-cycle variation, creating a glottal cycle as in (A), or could highlight variation.

In the disordered voice, irregularities are more frequent and/or more pronounced, and unfortunately may be missed by videostroboscopic sampling, making it critical that the clinician observe over long samples of phonation. In (C) hypofunctional vocal folds show a long open phase and touch closure. In (D) hyperfunctional cycles show a long closed phase and small amplitude of movement.

(continued)

Figure 4–6 (continued)

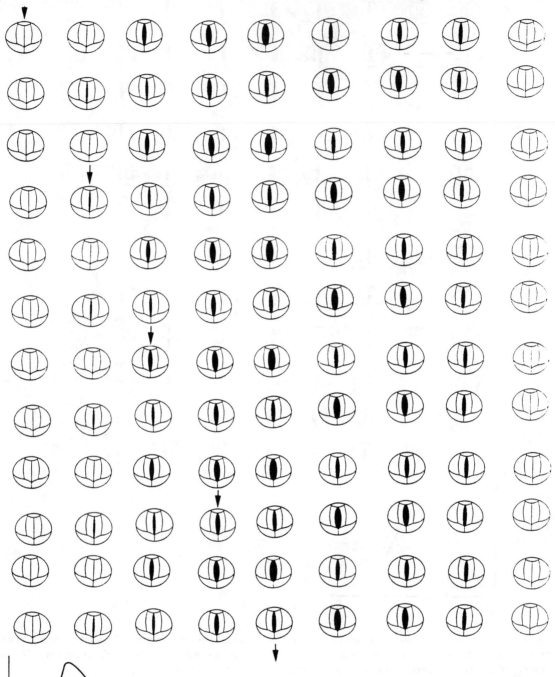

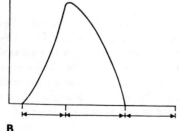

B

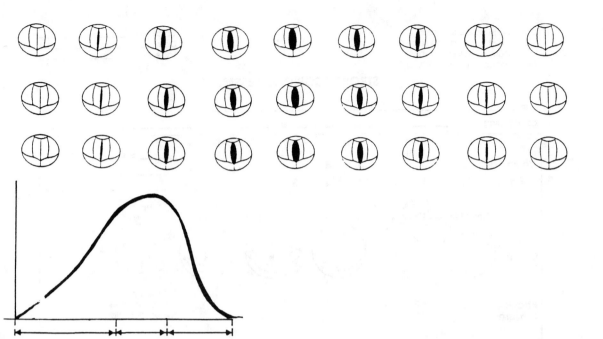

C

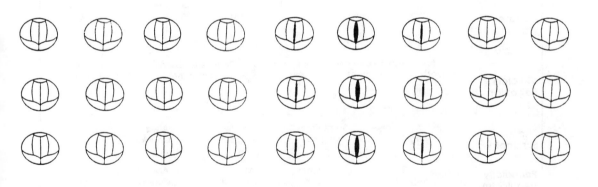

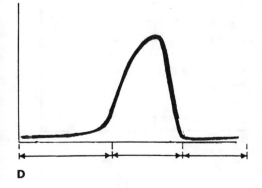

D

Chart no._____
Date:_____
Tape no. _____

STROBOSCOPIC ASSESSMENT

Name:_____ (M or F)   Age: _____

Clinical Diagnosis_____

		Smooth Straight				Rough Irregular	**COMMENTS**
Voice Fold	R	1	2	3	4	5	FO _____ SPL:_____
Edge	L	1	2	3	4	5	Voice quality_____

	Complete	Ant. Chink	Irreg.	Bowing	Post. Chink	Hour-glass	In-complete
Glottic Closure							

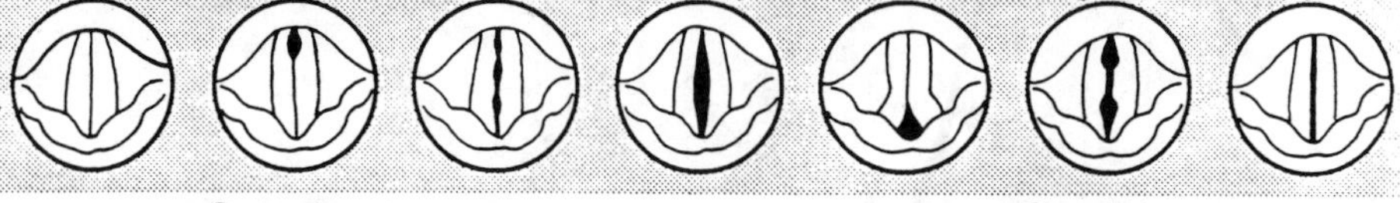

	Open phase predominates (whisper)		Normal		Closed phase predominates (hyperadduction)
Phase Closure	1	2	3	4	5

	Equal	R. lower	L. lower	Questionable
Vertical level vf approx.	1	2	3	4

		Normal	Slightly Decreased	Moderately Decreased	Severely Decreased	No Visible Movement
Amplitude	R	1	2	3	4	5
	L	1	2	3	4	5

		Normal	Slightly Decreased	Moderately Decreased	Severely Decreased	Absent
Mucosal Wave	R	1	2	3	4	5
	L	1	2	3	4	5

		Always fully present	Partial absence sometimes	Partial absence always	Complete absence sometimes	Complete absence always
Vibratory Behavior	R	1	2	3	4	5
	L	1	2	3	4	5

	Regular	Sometimes Irregular	Mostly Irregular	Always Irregular
Phase Symmetry	1	2	3	4

	Regular	Sometimes Irregular	Mostly Irregular	Always Irregular
Periodicity (regularity)	1	2	3	4

Ventricular Folds: Symmetry of movement: 1. R>L   2. L>R   3. Equal

Movement:	Normal	Sl. Compress	Mod. Compress	Full Compress
	1	2	3	4

Arytenoids: Symmetry of movement: 1. R>L   2. L>R   3. Equal

Movement:	Normal	Fair	Poor
	1	2	3

Hyperfunction: 1. not present   2. sometimes present   3. always present

Figure 4–7. Stroboscopic assessment form.

A stroboscopic evaluation was completed during phonation of the sustained vowel /i/ using a rigid endoscope. The vowel was produced at normal pitch (240 Hz) and loudness level (68 dB re: 002 dynes/cm²), at a high pitch (440 Hz), and during loud phonation (89 dB). Vocal fold movement was observed to be asymmetrical during all three vowel production conditions. The amplitude of vibration was small during normal pitch and loudness and increased only slightly during loud phonation. The amplitude appeared to be normal during the high pitch productions when it is expected to be small. Aperiodicity was present throughout phonation as was evidenced by visible motion during the "beat off" condition. An adynamic segment approximately 2–3 mm long beginning 1–2 mm from the left anterior commissure was noted. The rest of the vocal cord has a mobile leading edge, but the motion is somewhat erratic, suggesting some mucosal edema. The right cord is bulkier than the left, and moves more slowly. At the junction of the anterior and middle thirds, there is an irregular mound of mucosa. This area is markedly hypodynamic when compared with the rest of the cord. At no time during the evaluation was any mucosal wave observed in this portion of the vocal fold. Glottal closure was incomplete.

Figure 4–8. Example of a narrative report.

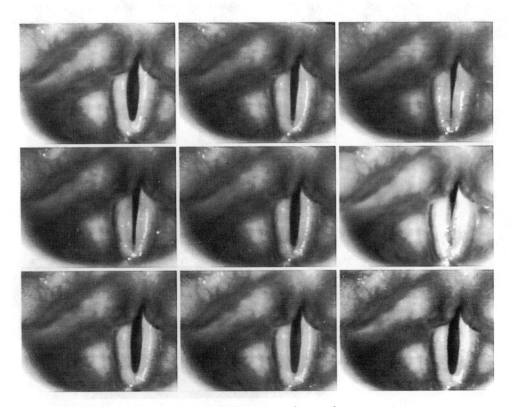

Figure 4–9. A video print of the type to be included in a patient's record.

Fees and Reimbursement

Fees should be based on a projected equipment depreciation cost per patient, clinician time required to perform the evaluation and generate the report, supplies such as tongue depressors and gauze, and indirect costs involved with space, scheduling patients, and record keeping. Special voice disorder clinics with a high patient volume are able to amortize equipment depreciation over a large base of patients and therefore may have somewhat lower expenses than clinics that see only five or six voice patients per week.

A summary of return on investment from stroboscopic examinations provided by Bruel and Kjaer instruments is contained in Figure 4–10. It is based on number of patients per week, fees, and cost of equipment. Details are presented in Appendix 4–2. These figures are derived from 1992 costs and could change based on economic conditions in the future.

Insurance coverage is variable. Usually, when the patient has taken the time to get appropriate referrals or has organic disease, when appropriate Current Procedural Terminology (CPT) Codes have been used, and when billing is through a physician, insurance coverage is 80% or greater. Coverage of nonorganic disease problems is more problematic. Medicare and Medicaid cover far less.

Not all carriers have a policy for reimbursement for stroboscopic examinations. This often necessitates written justification for the services provided from the examining clinician. The probability of getting full coverage is increased when the explanation includes information describing the procedure and the equipment needed to execute it, the purpose of the procedure, the frequency with which the procedure is done, and the range of charges levied in the examiner's own geographical region and across the nation. A useful request for payment for videoendostroboscopic evaluation was generated by the staff at the Phonometric Laboratory in Syracuse, State University of New York (SUNY) (Appendix 4–3).

A proposal for insurance coverage has been developed by Stone and Lingeman (1987) (Appendix 4–4). This proposal serves as a model for presenting rationale for coverage to different carriers. Clinicians can help facilitate coverage by submitting proposals explaining the services, costs, and procedures similar to the proposal developed by Stone.

All the foregoing suggestions are designed simply as aids to the stroboscopist. The stroboscope is but an additional clinical tool for acquiring data on vocal function and/or pathology. When data have been generated through proper clinical procedures, the task of judging patients' vibratory patterns and interpreting their meanings falls to the examiner.

Return on Investment from Stroboscopic Examinations

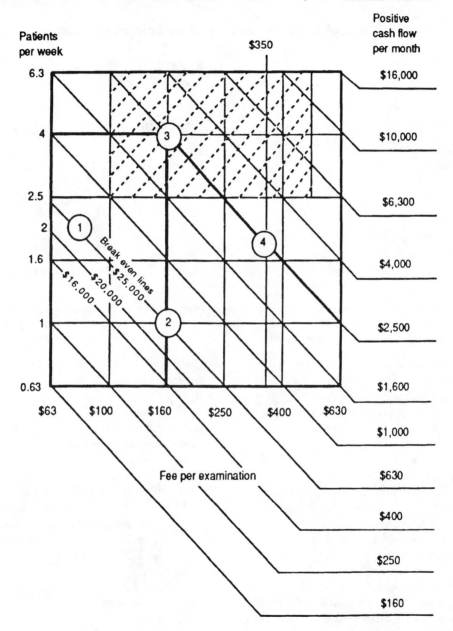

Figure 4–10. Return on investment from stroboscopic examinations. The break-even lines for three different priced instruments ($16,000, $20,000, and $25,000) are found on the diagonal lines in the lower left hand corner of the chart. Points (1) and (2) show that a system purchased at $25,000 is completely paid for with two patients per week and a $80.00 fee, or one patient per week and a $160.00 fee. Other points on the line provide other possible combinations. This diagram of equipment depreciation does not include replacement of stroboscopic bulbs or other expenses related to personnel and indirect costs, or post-1993 financial condition changes.

APPENDIX 4–1

Protocol for Laryngeal Stroboscopic Evaluation[1]

RE: (Name)   EXAM DATE

(Address)   Referral Source

(City, St. ZIP)   Address

(Phone)   City, St. ZIP

(Age)   Phone

Clinician   Referral Dx.:

Last/next laryngologist appointment:

Voice Problem (onset and characteristics):

(NAME) was seen pursuant to difficulties with voice production upon referral by _____. Laryngeal function was examined and the results are listed below.

(Check, or circle the numerals, or before the numerals of an appropriate response — write: "2" for right-sided, "3" for bilateral, "4" for left-sided observations, "U" for items you are uncertain about or "NA" for items not attended to during the exam.)

The examination was conducted using
1   standard laryngeal mirror methodology
2   rigid fiberscopic methodology
3   flexible fiberscopic methodology
4   using a consant light source
5   using stroboscopic illumination
6   with anesthesia
7   without anesthesia.

The vocalization task upon which most of the results are based involved a loudness level that was
8   quiet to conversational
9   conversational to loud

during production of
10   a sustained vowel
11   connected speech.

The major part of the examination involved the patient's use of a fundamental frequency around _____ Hz. Periodicity of the glottal tone
12   did
13   did not

permit detailed examination of vocal fold vibration via stroboscopy.

Confidence in the results should be influenced by the facts that the patient
14   did
15   did not

expose the larynx long enough to make all the desired observations without gagging (but/and) the exam
16   was completed
17   was aborted.

Views of the larynx and vocal folds
18   were obtained of the entire laryngeal anatomy
19   were obtained for only a portion of the laryngeal anatomy. (If 19, identify where below.)

Video-taped documentation
20   was
21   was not

satisfactory in terms of
22   focus
23   lighting
24   both focus and lighting.

[1] From Stone, R. E. (Ed), Jr. (1986). *Protocol for laryngeal stroboscopic evaluation.* Unpublished manuscript. Vanderbilt University, Nashville, TN, with permission.

ANATOMY

The view of the larynx *excluding the vocal folds* was unremarkable in terms of

25 shape
26 size
27 mucosal color
28 mucosal topography
29 all of the above

(but) notable in terms of

30 shape
31 size
32 mucosal color
33 mucosal topography.

Specifically, shape of the larynx was remarkable with the presence of

34 crossed arytenoids
35 post-interarytenoid prominence
36 subglottal interarytenoid tissue redundancy
37 large false fold(s)
38 extreme curvature of epiglottis
39 flattening of epiglottis
40 asymmetry of epiglottis

Abnormal laryngeal

41 size
42 mucosal color and/or
43 mucosal topography

can be described as:

44 (comment)

Mucus on the vocal folds appeared

45 appropriate in amount
46 decreased in amount

as indicated by a(an) (paucity/abundance) of light reflexes.

Pooling on the folds was

47 minimal
48 significant

(and/but) stranding of mucus across the glottis was

49 minimal
50 significant.

Appearance of the *vocal folds* seemed

51 unremarkable (If this choice is appropriate go to number 101.)

52 noteworthy (If this choice is appropriate, any written report should identify items below that were unremarkable by default as suggested by absence of notations.)

in terms of

53 length of the fold
54 lateral cord thickness
55 vertical cord thickness
56 position and/or movements of the fold during respiration or for phonation
57 mucosal color of the fold
58 vascularity of the fold
59 general shape of vocal fold
60 mucosal topography
61 all of the above
62 The unusal _____ (i.e., length, thickness, positions, mucosal color, vascularity, and/or vocal fold shape) took on the general characteristic(s) of:
(indicate below)

The location of the irregularity of the mucus membrane seemed centered at or near the

63 anterior commissure
64 anterior one-third of the fold
65 junction of the first and second third of the fold
66 middle third of the fold
67 posterior third of the fold
68 posterior commissure

on the

69 upper surface of the cord
70 glottal surface of the cord
71 subglottal surface of the cord.

The lateral dimension of the surface irregularity appeared to be

72 less than 25% of the fold's width
73 approximately 25% of the fold's width
74 between 25% and 50% of the fold's width
75 approximately 50% of the fold's width
76 approximately 100% or more of the fold's width

and anterior/posteriorly was

77 less than 25% of the fold's width
78 approximately 25% of the fold's width
79 between 25% and 50% of the fold's width

80   approximately 50% of the fold's width
81   approximately 100% or more of the fold's width.

The irregularity of the mucous membrane on the fold(s) appeared

82   translucent
83   opaque
84   white
85   red
86   bluish-gray
87   yellowish-brown
88   other color _____ ,
89   hard and organized
90   soft and unorganized
91   smooth surfaced
92   rough surfaced
93   sessile
94   pedunculated
95   pointed
96   rounded
97   square shouldered
98   elliptical
99   other _____ .

VOCAL CORD PHYSIOLOGY
(STROBOSCOPY EXAM)

Stroboscopic examination
100   also showed
101   failed to show

this mucus membrane irregularity on the fold(s).
SYMMETRY of glottal activity studied stroboscopically

102   invariably was
103   most of the time was
104   was not always
105   never was

observed using stroboscopy.
>>>If 102 or 103 is the appropriate choice, go to AMPLITUDE section below<<<
Asymmetry was observed in terms of

106   anterior deviation of the glottis
107   (the indicated) fold was higher than the other
108   vertical movement of (indicated) fold preceded the other
109   lateral movement of (indicated) fold preceded and/or was (less/greater), than the other.

AMPLITUDE of lateral movement of the (indicated) fold(s), in modal register, which contributes to symmetry seemed

110   unremarkable
111   great
112   small
113   absent

on

114   a consistent basis
115   an inconsistent basis
116   other comments:

PERIODICITY of glottal activity seemed

117   regular
118   irregular
119   on a consistent basis
120   on an inconsistent basis.

The MUCOSAL WAVE ACTION of the superior surface of the (indicated) vocal fold(s) during modal register phonations appeared

121   normal
122   great
123   small
124   absent

on

125   a consistent basis
126   an inconsistent basis.

The different-than-normal mucous membrane undulations were most notable on the fold(s) at

127   the anterior third
128   the junction of the anterior and middle thirds of the fold
129   the middle third of the fold.
130   throughout the entire length of the fold.

CLOSURE of the glottis was complete

131   all the time
132   some of the time

was incomplete

133   all the time
134   some of the time

and revealed a(an)

135   posterior chink
136   variable pattern of where the glottal opening was located
137   spindle or elliptical-shaped opening

138 incompetence glottal slit for most of the length
139 hour-glass shape
140 anterior chink
141 other _____ .

COMMENTS

142

INTERPRETATION

These findings suggest
143 unremarkable structure and/or vibratory motion of the vocal folds.
144 notable anatomy and/or vibratory motion of the vocal folds.
The ASYMMETRY may best be explained by
145 abnormal position of the vocal folds
146 abnormal shape of the vocal folds
147 altered mass of the (indicated) vocal folds
148 altered tension of the (indicated) fold
149 altered elasticity and viscosity of the (indicated) folds
150 inadequate training or failure to benefit from vocal training
151 inexplicable causes.
ABNORMAL AMPLITUDE of vocal fold excursions seems attributable to
152 a shortened vibratory portion of the glottis
153 altered stiffness of the affected fold
154 altered mass of the affected fold
155 decreased subglottal pressure during phonation
156 unknown factors.
PERIODICITY of cord activity might be due to unequal
157 position
158 shape
159 mass
160 tension
161 elasticity and viscosity between the two cords
162 inconsistent neuromuscular control
163 inconsistent subglottal pressure
164 unknown factors.

The aberration of the MUCOSAL WAVE may best be explained by
165 stiffened mucosa
166 submucosal abnormality
167 unknown causes.
The incomplete GLOTTAL CLOSURE seemingly is explained by
168 impaired adduction
169 (bowing of, or divot in) the glottal margin(s)
170 an interposed excrescence
171 non-homogeneous mucosal elasticity and viscosity
of the (indicated) vocal fold(s).
172 unknown factors.

From these observations and interpretations one might ascribe the voice and laryngeal differences to: (identify the most probable disruptive factor(s) below)

_____ . Alternately, other considerations such as

_____

might be reasonably entertained.

POTENTIAL DISRUPTIVE FACTORS

.100 Dysplasia
.110   Webbing of the vocal folds
.120   Vocal fold sulci
.130   Bowed folds

.200 Non-malignant lesion
.210   Papillomatosis
.220   Keratosis and leukoplakia
.230   Polyps (not due to vocal abuse)
.240   Polyps and nodules (due to vocal abuse)
.250   Contact ulcers and/or intubation Granulomas
.260   Cysts, laryngoceles, amyloidosis, or lipoid proteinosis
.270   Vocal cord thickening

.300 Malignant lesion

.400 Varicosity, hemorrhage, inflammation (laryngitis)

.500	Trauma		.721	Thyroid
.510	Dislocations		.722	Parathyroid
.520	Stenosis		.723	Functional sicca or sicca components of other syndromes
.530	Scarring			

.500   Trauma
.510   Dislocations
.520   Stenosis
.530   Scarring

.600   Paralysis
.610   Recurrent N. paralysis
.620   Superior N. paralysis
.630   CNS paralysis
.640   Motor end plate disorder or other myopathies

.700   Hormonal
.710   Gonadal including menstruational and menopausal
.720   Other endocrine and metabolic

.721   Thyroid
.722   Parathyroid
.723   Functional sicca or sicca components of other syndromes

.800   Unhygienic voice production and/or laryngel condition
.810   Vocal abuse
.820   Vocal fatigue

.900   Misuse (Hyperkinetic dysphonia, muscular tension dysphonia)
.910   Spastic dysphonia
.920   Dysphonia plica ventricularis
.997   Deferred opinion
.998   No factors seem related

APPENDIX 4–2

Returns on Investment for Using Videostroboscopy of the Larynx by Brüel & Kjaer Instruments, Inc.[1]

"The larynx stroboscope is the single most important instrument procurement after basic instruments," say all otolaryngologists who have become experienced with its use. They need the stroboscope since it adds significantly to the accuracy of many of their diagnoses. The addition of video camera and recording fulfills documentation and communication needs.

"Yes, but how can we bear the cost of such an instrument," is the response of some physicians who have not yet accepted the need for high quality electronic instrumentation in their practice.

In otolaryngology, as in other fields, physicians have started to use sophisticated instrumentation because it adds greatly to their diagnostic capabilities, and thereby to the overall performance of their office.

Investment Needs for Videostroboscopy (Because of fluctuating economic conditions, money amounts are likely to change.)

The price for a total system may be held as low as $25,000, of which the basic stroboscope is only about $17,000 and video equipment about $4,000.

If cash flow is a vital concern, the system may be leased. The outlay for a 5-year lease, even with 4-month deferred payments, would be less than:

Basic stroboscope	$17,000; 5 years @ $400/month
Stroboscope w/video	$21,000; 5 years @ $500/month
Stroboscope w/video & endoscope	$25,000; 5 years @ $600/month

Cashflow for Using Videostroboscopy

Let us not forget that a new technique also provides new remuneration. Comparing outlay with positive cash flow, we can construct the attached diagram (logarithmic scales) (see Figure 4–10).

The number of patients per week (0.6 to 6.3 or 2.5 to 25 per month) is given on the left vertical scale.

The fee per stroboscopic examination ($63 to $630) is given on the horizontal scale; $350 per examination has been proposed in Indiana

The figures in the right hand column are the monthly gross revenues for any given combination of number of patients per week and fee per examination.

Break-Even Calculations

The break-even lines for three purchase options are given by the three labeled diagonal lines in the lower left corner of the chart. Points (1) and (2) show that even a total system purchase at $25,000 is completely paid for

[1] Reprinted courtesy of Brüel & Kjaer Instruments, Inc.

with two patients per week and an $80 fee, or one patient per week and a $160 fee. Other points on the line provide other possible combinations. By choosing a lease with deferred payments (4 months), a positive cash flow may be developed before payments are commenced.

Returns on Investment

Let us take a look at the possible return by the use of videostroboscopy. As an example, let us assume the combination of four patients per week at a fee schedule of $160 per exam (Point 3) or less than two patients per week at the suggested $350 (Point 4).

Straight purchase may be a preferable option depending on tax ramifications, with payback in 10 months (for a $25,000 purchase price).

APPENDIX 4-3

Sample Request For Payment [1]

To Whom It May Concern:

Over the past two years in excess of 50 centers throughout the United States that are recognized for their leadership in the diagnosis and treatment of laryngeal disorders have incorporated the use of new procedures into their practice. These procedures involve Videoendostroboscopy (Videostroboendoscopy, Laryngostroboscopy, Videolaryngostroboscopy, Phonostroboscopy) to document laryngeal anatomy, pathology, and vocal fold activity before and after behavioral/medical/surgical treatment and to aid in the diagnosis of laryngeal pathology and dysfunction. For all indications, fees that are charged range up to $_____ per evaluation. The median fee is $_____, and the mode appears to be approximately $475.

Our fee schedule is based upon a projected equipment depreciation cost per patient, clinician time required to perform the evaluation, and indirect cost involved with scheduling patients, materials, typing, etc. Our estimates are less than the average fees for the country, partly because of the estimated high volume of patients we anticipate.

The endoscopic procedures involve viewing the larynx with either a rigid fiberoptic endoscope or a flexible fiberoptic endoscope. Use of the rigid scope generally requires no anesthesia as it is placed intraorally. The flexible scope requires anesthetization of the nasal passages and hypopharynx. When endoscopy is videotaped, special professional quality equipment is used with specialized lighting source that provides continuous light. Stroboscopy involves the use of intermittent light activated by the action of the vocal folds involving specialized acoustic signal-processing and electronics as well as a unique light source. It enables viewing the vocal folds in slow motion for studying details of vibratory motion that cannot be appreciated otherwise.

[1] From Colton, R., Casper, J., Brewer, D., Woo, P., and Bless, D. H. (1991, November). Stroboscopic evaluation of the larynx. Workshop. American Speech-Language-Hearing Association National Convention, Atlanta, GA, with permission.

APPENDIX 4–4

Abbreviated Explanation and Justification of Videoendoscopy and Videostroboscopy Submitted in Request for Reimbursement of Fees[1]

Standard Medical Practices include the examination of patients' larynges when they present themselves with vocal complaints or demonstrate dysphonia. The oldest technique for such examination is identified as a "mirror exam," or indirect examination. More recently flexible and/or rigid fiberoptic endoscopes have been used. In a few centers and clinics the newer techniques are augmented by video recording the images for evaluation by repeated playback. This *videoendoscopy* embodies the benefit of graphic documentation of patient's laryngeal anatomy that is unparalleled by any other method in terms of efficacy, cost, and clinician time.

Videostroboscopy is a technique that allows viewing not only detailed anatomy (permitted by techniques previously mentioned) but also the patient's physiology of phonation. This is accomplished by procedures and equipment that make the visual images of the vocal folds (vibrating too rapidly to be seen by the unaided eye) to appear as if seen "in stop action or in slow motion." Thus, physiological aberrations can be appreciated that cannot be seen by any other economical way. The video recordings benefit evaluation by the option of repeated playback.

These newer video-aided techniques result in greater confidence of diagnosis and opportunity to form diagnoses where without such techniques no diagnosis or misdiagnosis might occur. Additionally, patient education is enhanced by showing the patient his/her own laryngeal images and, therefore, patient compliance often is increased. Viewing recordings that are made repeatedly over time aids in evaluation of changes in laryngeal status and, therefore, can be a guide to the need to change therapeutic efforts or to continue them. This technique represents the only suitable avenue to assessing client's visible changes in physiology as a function of therapy. It, then, is indispensable for rendering valid accountability.

Characteristics of vocal fold vibration determine the major attributes of voice. These include: pitch (correlated with fundamental frequency); loudness (correlated with intensity); and, to a large extent, quality (correlated with acoustic spectra). Abnormal vocal fold vibration contributes to the existence of aberrant voice characteristics that may lead to a diagnosis of dysphonia. Abnormal vibration patterns are expected in the presence of laryngeal pathology but also may occur as a result of misuse of normal structures. Thus, evaluation of dysphonia currently employs both perceptual judgments made by a clinician and visual examination of laryngeal anatomy and laryngeal function by mirror examination, by endoscopic procedures (rigid endoscopy, flexible fiberendoscopy), or by direct observation in a procedure room. There are, however, clinical instances in which dysphonia cannot be explained by results of such visual examination. Some parts of the larynx move faster than what can be visually perceived. Furthermore, the "real time" observations cannot be played back for reconsideration. Therefore, etiology of dysphonia for some patients is undetermined. For others, dysphonia is attributed to erroneous etiological factors. Both missed diagnoses and misdiagnoses lead to misdirected therapeutic interventions and involve unnecessary patient costs and detain instatement of appropriate therapeutics.

To overcome such problems, a stroboscopic technique of laryngeal examination with suitable refinements recently has been reintroduced to the fields of laryngology and speech pathology. Used in conjunction with video recordings, a permanent videostroboscopic record can be obtained. When studied by trained observers, the records aid detection of pathology of the vocal folds that would be made by traditional observation methods but with the advantage of being able to make additional observations of

[1] From Stone, R. E. (Ed), Jr., and Lingeman, Raleigh E. (1986). *A proposal for insurance coverage of laryngeal videoendoscopic and videostroboscopic examinations.* Unpublished manuscript, Indiana University School of Medicine, Department of Otolaryngology-Head and Neck Surgery, Indianapolis, with permission.

structure and function of the cords that cannot be assessed with standard evaluations. This technique, new to the battery of clinical tools, has the advantage of recording the observations photographically. These, when compared over time with earlier records of a given patient, permit evaluation of the remission of a person's laryngeal pathology and laryngeal malfunction that might be expected to occur with a given therapeutic approach. Thus, new procedures for evaluating clinical accountability of intervention are added to the services of the health care provider. This proposal overviews the technique, equipment, and personnel that might be involved in laryngeal stroboscopy, suggests minimal standards of a complete examination, and proposes reimbursement of fees for services.

From the array of sound producing instruments there is not one that demonstrates greater flexibility and variety than the human voice. Furthermore, it provides a window to the health, mind, body and soul (of) its user, be he just a few seconds into earthly life or just a few moments from his eternal life.

Background Information

Vibration of the vocal folds is the crucial event necessary for voice production. The vibratory pattern of the vocal folds can be described with respect to various parameters including:

1. the repetition rate of the vibration,
2. the regularity or periodicity in successive vibrations,
3. symmetry of motion between the two vocal folds,
4. uniformity or homogeneity in the movement of different points within each vocal fold,
5. glottal closure during vibration,
6. amplitude of vocal fold motion,
7. wave which travels on the mucosa covering the folds, and
8. contact area and shape between the two vocal folds (modified from Hirano, 1981).

Yet, most of these parameters cannot be analyzed apart from the use of ultra-high-speed-photography (which is too inefficient and costly for clinical use) or by stroboscopic techniques (which heretofore have barely provided adequate light).

Laryngeal stroboscopy first came into use as a means of observing the normal vibration of the vocal folds

nearly 100 years ago. In the early stages, mechanical devices were used to obtain an intermittent source of light. It was, therefore, difficult to examine pathological vibrations with associated irregular cycle-to-cycle variations. A strobo-light bulb activated by the vibration of the vocal folds came into existence in the 1950s (Beck & Schönharl, 1954; Timcke, 1956a, b). Schönharl (1960b) pioneered the inclusion of stroboscopy in laryngological practice in Europe where it has received continuing popularity. In the United States, interest in laryngology and stroboscopy has yet to parallel that in Europe but since the introduction of the new version of the Brüel and Kjaer Stroboscope (1984) stroboscopy has received increasing interest and use.

Technique

Laryngeal stroboscopy permits observation of the larynx when it is illuminated by intermittent flashes of light which are synchronous with the vibratory cycles of the vocal folds or slightly delayed from flash to flash. The source of the trigger signal for the light flashes is the subject's voice. When the flashes are emitted at the same frequency as that of the vocal fold vibration at an identical point in successive vibratory cycles, a sharp and clear "stop action" image of the vocal folds is observed. A slow motion effect is produced when the flashes are emitted at frequencies slightly different (to an extent controlled by the examiner) than the frequency of vocal fold vibration. Stroboscopy does not show fine details of each vibratory cycle, but it demonstrates a vibratory pattern based upon visualization of sequential parts of rapidly occurring cyclic events making the events appear as a slowly occurring behavior.

This instrumentation also permits viewing the larynx with a light source that is constant (not dependent upon vocal fold vibration). With either of the two light sources video recordings can be made by attaching a video camera on the laryngeal mirror or endoscope used in conjunction with the stroboscope. Thus, traditional laryngeal examination can be performed, and as with stroboscopy, may be conducted with or without video recording. Since both procedures are so similar and both are done when stroboscopy is performed, the term "laryngeal videoendoscopy/videostroboscopic" has been coined for this proposal.

Instrumentation

The equipment used in this procedure consists of three parts: Laryngeal viewing systems, Light source and controls and Visual recording (documentation) systems. Views of the larynx may be obtained using a standard laryngeal mirror, rigid endoscopes, or flexible fiberoptic endoscopes which are standard equipment in most voice clinics and cost upwards to $3,000.

The light source and control system involves halogen or xenon lamps which are activated in various ways. First a constant light is usually activated by the examiner for obtaining a general laryngeal exam. Light is transmitted from the stroboscopic unit to the laryngeal mirror or endoscope through a flexible fiberoptic cable. When vibratory motion of the cords is to be examined, the patient is fitted with a throat microphone. The output of the microphone is led to special electronic equipment in the stroboscopic unit which turns on and off the light that is led to the viewing instrument to illuminate the larynx. These flashes may be adjusted by the examiner to illuminate the larynx at any repeated position of the cords during successive vibratory cycles to obtain a "static" view of the vocal folds. By slowly adjusting the point of the vibratory cycle at which the larynx is illuminated, "slow motion" impressions of the cord activity can be obtained. Cost of this portion of the system begins at $17,000.

Documenting that which is observed on video tape involves attaching a video camera (up to $8,000) to an endoscope and viewing the laryngeal behaviors on a monitor (up to $800) for selection of behaviors to be recorded using a VCR (up to $25,000). Some units (Brüel and Kjaer, for example), also, have provision for obtaining 35 mm still pictures. The camera is adapted to fit onto the endoscope and is triggered during stroboscopic examination. (Camera and accessories cost approximately $1,000.)

Benefits

It's common knowledge in the areas of phonatory research and theory that differences in parameters of vocal fold vibration exist between production of normal and abnormal (dysphonia) voice production. When the differences are known to be present in a patient with laryngeal complaints a clinician is inclined to ascribe the dysphonia to organic etiology and follow a particular course of intervention. When parameters cannot be studied or when changes in them are not perceived, an associated dysphonia erroneously might be ascribed to non-organic etiology with another course of intervention being recommended. Inadequate and missed diagnoses often leads to formulation of a favorable prognosis for a patient and might encourage unsuccessful and unnecessary prolongation of behavioral or psychiatric based therapy. Similarly, missed diagnosis also might unnecessarily lead to postponement of needed intervention of medical/surgical natures.

Stroboscopy provides a means of decreasing the incidence of erroneous diagnoses and invalid treatment plans. Three 35mm still pictures of a subject's vocal folds were examined. In the first photograph, five out of five laryngologists felt that there was evidence suggestive of a vocal cord nodule and recommended surgical removal. Photograph number 2 was interpreted as representing leukoplakia and the physicians all suggested that a biopsy be conducted. The third photograph was interpreted as a probable polyp by two laryngologists who recommended confirmation via direct laryngoscopy. The remaining three laryngologists felt the excrescence was probably a vocal cord cyst and recommended surgical removal. It is pointed out, however, that the laryngologists' opinions were elicited without presenting any patient history and without opportunity for repeated examination which each physician indicated would be desirable, preferably at another appointment. When the larynx was examined by stroboscopic procedures, each of the images was observed; *but* were found to be transitory collections of mucous in a normal larynx.

Had the subject been an actual patient who could offer only a brief view of her larynx in a clinic without a stroboscope, additional expenses for re-examination or unnecessary expenses for inappropriate treatment assuredly would have been incurred. Stroboscopy would have avoided direct patient and/or third-party expenses.

Being able to study the various parameters of vocal fold vibration and to be influenced by them in forming diagnoses may also benefit earlier detection of disease, earlier treatment and less patient cost with improved results. Even with the undesirable attributes of earlier stroboscopes, Luchsinger and Arnold (1965, p. 56) reported three cases in which stroboscopy was beneficial.

> two patients with chronic vocal complaints were observed with ordinary laryngoscopy, both showed the minor findings of reddening and dryness of the normally moveable vocal cords. Stroboscopy, however, revealed vibratory immobility of one cord, which suggested an organic unilateral lesion. Subsequent biopsy led to the diagnosis of early carcinoma. Both patients were treated successfully by cordectomy. In a third case, stroboscopy showed vibratory immobility of one cord. Sometime later, granulomatous vegetations became visible (on) ordinary laryngoscopy, slightly below the affected vocal cord.

Failure to utilize the benefits of this new laryngeal examination technique not only outdates a clinician's standard operating procedures but increases the possibility of medical legal action for failure to practice the best available delivery of services. It would be analogous to an otologist's practicing without using audiometrics. When videostroboscopy that is now available is not used, an argument for inadequate practice might be based upon failure to utilize all possible diagnostic capabilities as well as ignoring the documentation benefits derived from adequate evaluation.

The advent of video tape recording, development of video cameras able to function with low level light sources and recent advances in light sources associated with the most modern laryngeal strobosopes constitute a major development in delivery of health care. Coupled with the use of video tape recording techniques, "stroboscopy has become an indispensable part of my office examination procedures" reports Dr. Robert Sataloff, a noted laryngologist in Philadelphia (personal communication, 1985). Stroboscopic Evaluation of the Larynx was the title of a workshop for speech pathologists and laryngologists held August, 1984, at the University of Wisconsin, and was repeated again September 1986, further illustrating that stroboscopy is a procedure that has a lasting attraction.

Other benefits from employing videostroboscopy can be anticipated:

- Improved patient compliance with recommendations brought about by patient education via video tapes revealing the laryngeal problem and its remission.
- More accurate information gleaned by allowing more than one specialist to view the vocal folds in motion at the same time. In addition, this technology permits repeated viewing at convenient times, improving office efficiency and patient services.
- Comparing vibratory patterns at different times including pre- and post-therapeutic examinations.
- Minimized chance for miscommunication with referral sources by visually sharing results of examination.
- Increased efficiency and lowered costs associated with seeking second opinions by sending video tapes to consultants rather than going to the expense of a patient's travel and office visit costs.
- Permits a means of rendering valid accountability of therapy.
- Provides for a patient (such as a touring vocalist with a recent voice complaint) to share with the consulting specialist a prior status of the larynx, if the patient obtained a video tape of a previous examination. Thus, the validity of interpretations of current findings might be enhanced. (Bless, D. M., Hirano, M., & Feder, R., 1984).

Proposed Minimal Standards of Stroboscopic Examination

Indications:

We propose that any of the following are patient indications for conducting videoendoscopy/videostroboscopy.

1. Abnormal voice characteristics or complaints about voice production without known organic etiology,
2. Abnormal voice characteristics following disruption in continuity of laryngeal mucosa (post surgery or trauma),
3. Suspicion of laryngeal paralysis/paresis,
4. Presence of laryngeal pathology.
5. The need to compare former videoendoscopic/videostroboscopic findings with current laryngeal status.

6. Abnormal voice characteristics which are incompatible with known laryngeal status

Observations:

Hirano (op cit) recommends stroboscopic examination results be described in terms of fundamental frequency of phonation which the patient used during the examination, bilateral symmetry of the vocal folds, regularity of the vibrations, glottal closure, amplitude of vocal cord excursion, mucosal wave, and non-vibrating portions of the cords. It may not be possible or desirable to evaluate all six of the above mentioned aspects in every assessment. Some patients, however, may not present views of the larynx enabling such observations. An examination worthy of full reimbursement should, we propose, result in at least three out of the six observations. We further propose that reported descriptions of laryngeal status and physiology and the interpretations thereof are to be made by either a Board-certified otolaryngologist or a licensed speech pathologist who meet further requirements listed under personnel qualifications, below.

The examination, "reading" the video tape and developing impressions, and report writing is expected to require approximately 1½ hours per patient.

Personnel Qualifications

Conduct of stroboscopic examinations is to be carried out by speech pathologists and/or laryngologists who equal or exceed the following:

1. Certified or are qualified to be certified by their respective professional national organizations,
2. Licensed to practice their respective professional duties in the state of _____,
3. Hold a Provider Number with Blue Cross,
4. Demonstrated expertise in laryngeal anatomy and in physiology of phonation,

5. Demonstrated expertise in the area of intervention in dysphonia, as evidenced, for example, by authorship of articles, chapters, books on intervention or participation on professional programs dealing with diagnosis and intervention.

Proposed Fee Schedule

Establishing "usual and customary fees" for this examination is impossible because of the paucity of centers performing such examination and the diversity of charges being assessed by centers that do provide such services. From our investigation it appears that fees range up to $1,000 per examination. A noted laryngologist in the Los Angeles area charges $475. We proposed a fee of $350.00 per evaluation.

References

Beck, J., & Schonharl, E. (1954). Ein neues mikrophongesteuertes Lichtblitz-Stroboskop. *HNO, 4,* 212–214.

Bless, D. M., Hirano, M., Feder, R. (1984). Stroboscopic Evaluation of the Larynx Workshop. [Madison].

Colton, R., Casper, J., Brewer, D., Woo, P., & Bless, D. M. (1991). Stroboscopic Evaluation of the Larynx Workshop. American Speech and Hearing Association, National Convention, Atlanta, GA.

Hirano, M. (1981a). *Clinical examination of voice.* Secaucus, NJ: Springer-Verlag.

Luchsinger, R., & Arnold, G. E. (1965). *Voice-speech-language.* (G. E. Arnold & E. R. Finkbeiner, Trans.) Belmont, CA: Wadsworth. (Original work 2nd. ed. published in 1959)

Schonharl, E. (1960a). *Die Stroboskopie in der praktischen Laryngologie.* Stuttgart: G. Thieme.

Timcke, R. (1956a). Die Synchron-Stroboskopie von menschlichen Stimmlippen bzw. äahnlichen Schallquellen und Messung der Öffnungszeit. *Z. F. Laryngology, Rhinology, and Otology, 35,* 331–335.

STUDY QUESTIONS

1. The choice of equipment used during strobo-scopic examination depends on:

   a. Purpose of testing and examiner.

   b. Available equipment.

   c. The patient's preference.

   d. a and b.

2. During stroboscopic examination with a rigid endoscope:

   a. 4% Lidocaine® spray should be administered.

   b. Examiner should protect the patient's teeth to avoid damage.

   c. Patient should be asked to phonate on /a/.

   d. None of the above.

3. Examination with a fiberscope:

   a. Requires anesthesia administered by the speech pathologist.

   b. Can be done by a team consisting of the physician and speech pathologist.

   c. Allows visualization of vocal fold vibration during connected speech.

   d. Is not a useful technique.

4. Which of the following statements is *true*?

   a. There is a set protocol for stroboscopic examination.

   b. The pathology dictates the protocol, thus the clinician must understand how the pathology affects the body-cover relationship.

5. Visual feedback can be useful:

   a. In cases of hyperfunction or laryngeal dyskinesia.

   b. In identifying behaviors that need to be modified.

   c. For long periods of time, making the patient depend on the visual image.

   d. a and b.

6. The following types of patient record keeping are suggested:

   a. Short narrative paragraph and videoprint.

   b. An elaborate checklist.

   c. Tape recording of the entire session.

   d. None of the above.

Judgment and Interpretation of Vibratory Pattern

Judging and interpreting observed vibratory patterns is the next step in using stroboscopy to address laryngeal problems. The vibratory pattern of vocal folds can be described and ascribed to pathologies with respect to the several major features or phenomena: frequency and periodicity, horizontal and vertical movement, and other features.

The examiner can use a standardized form to record stroboscopic findings (see Chapter 4, Appendix 4–1). This chapter takes the examiner through each of the parameters listed above, with guidelines for judging those features and interpreting their implications.

FUNDAMENTAL FREQUENCY AND PERIODICITY

Fundamental Frequency (F₀)

Judgment and Description

The fundamental frequency is read in Hz on the F_0 indicator of the stroboscope. When it varies dur-

ing the examination, the range of the variation should be described.

Interpretation

As it is well-known that the pattern of vocal fold vibration varies with the fundamental frequency being produced, it is imperative that clinicians interpreting the data take into account the variables that might influence it. The following tendencies are relevant in interpreting the data. The examples provided do not necessarily occur in all instances.

The Stiffer the Vocal Fold Tissue, the Greater the Fundamental Frequency. An increase in the activity of the cricothyroid muscle stretches and stiffens the vocal fold tissue, resulting in a high fundamental frequency. This is an example of physiological variation. As pathological examples, scar formation of the vocal fold and sulcus vocalis tend to cause an increase in fundamental frequency.

The Shorter the Vibrating Portion of the Vocal Fold, the Greater the Fundamental Fre-

quency. In physiological variations, the fundamental frequency is usually higher in children than in adults and higher in female adults than males. Laryngeal web is a pathological example. With the occurrence of a web, the vibrating portion is shortened, resulting in a high fundamental frequency.

The Greater the Mass of the Vocal Fold, the Smaller the Fundamental Frequency. In the presence of a polyp or of Reinke's edema, the fundamental frequency tends to be low.

The Greater the Subglottal Pressure, the Greater the Fundamental Frequency. The influence of the subglottal pressure on the fundamental frequency is rather small and clinically not very important. The rate is 2–4 Hz/cm H_2O for modal voice and 7–10 Hz/cm H_2O for falsetto (Hirano, Vennard, & Ohala, 1970).

Periodicity

Judgment and Description

Periodicity is based on the regularity of successive apparent cycles of vocal fold vibration. "Periodic" vibration is considered to be uniform in amplitude and time; "aperiodic" vibration can vary in either or both (Figure 5–1).

The periodicity of a patient's voice can be determined by switching the beat frequency regulator on the stroboscopic generator from the beat "on" (slow motion) to the beat "off" (stop motion) position while the subject phonates. When the beat frequency is "off," periodic vocal fold vibration is reflected as a static image. Conversely, aperiodicity appears as observable movement of the vocal folds in the beat "off" state. (See also Chapter 3, section "Apparent Motion and Aperiodic Vibration.") Observations are rated three ways:

Regular (periodic). Image in the beat "off" state is static.

Irregular (aperiodic). Successive cycles of vibration appear irregular and no observable movement of the vocal folds is noted in the beat "off" state.

Inconsistent. The vibratory pattern is sometimes regular and sometimes irregular.

Interpretation

Maintenance of periodic vibrations of a vibrator calls for a steady balance between the mechanical properties of the vibrator — in other words, the vocal fold — and the force applied to the vibrator — for example, the pulmonary pressure. The following conditions can impair this balance and result in aperiodic or irregular vibrations.

Asymmetry. Marked asymmetry in the mechanical properties of the vocal folds can be caused by unilateral recurrent laryngeal nerve paralysis, unilateral polyp, or unilateral carcinoma.

Interference with Homogeneity. Marked interference with the homogeneity of the vocal fold(s) can be caused by a small cyst or a small carcinoma.

Flaccidity. Abnormally flaccid or pliable tissue can be caused by severe recurrent laryngeal nerve paralysis or an edematous lesion.

Unsteady Tonus. Incapability of maintaining a steady tonus of the laryngeal muscles can be caused by spastic dysphonia or other neuromuscular disease.

Inconsistent Force. Incapability of exhaling air from the lungs with a consistent force can be caused by neuromuscular diseases or pulmonary diseases.

HORIZONTAL AND VERTICAL MOVEMENTS

Amplitude of Horizontal (Latero-Medial) Excursion

Judgment and Description

Amplitude is defined as the extent of horizontal (latero-medial) excursion of the vocal folds during vibration. Each vocal fold is rated independently for

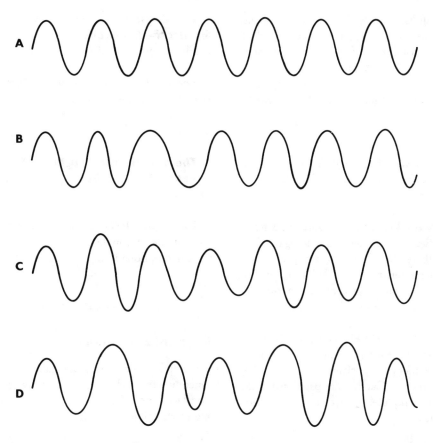

Figure 5–1. Glottal waveforms illustrate periodic and aperiodic vibration. (A) Waveform from one period to the next is uniform in amplitude and time and therefore considered to be periodic; (B) Waveform is the same in amplitude but varies in time and is therefore considered to have jitter; (C) Waveform is uniform in time but aperiodic in amplitude and thus has jitter; and (D) Waveform is aperiodic, varying from one cycle to the next both in time and in amplitude.

this parameter. Amplitude ratings are made on a four-point equal-appearing intervals scale.

Zero. No horizontal excursion of the vocal fold is observed.

Small. Horizontal excursion of the vocal fold is smaller than normal.

Normal. Horizontal excursion is within the normal range.

Great. Horizontal excursion of the vocal fold is greater than normal.

The amplitude of the two vocal folds should be compared and the findings should be described as "Right > Left," "Right = Left," or "Right < Left."

The "normal range" means the range of the amplitude for the "habitual pitch and habitual loudness" in typical subjects. The absolute amplitude is contingent on the size of the vocal folds; thus, it tends to be larger for adults. Usually, the amplitude of the horizontal excursion is approximately one-third of the width of the visible part of the vocal fold in normal subjects (Figure 5–2). At present, the assessment of the amplitude is made subjectively. Objective quantification awaits further technical developments.

Interpretation

Several general rules affect amplitude of vibration. Each of these can be exemplified by physiological or pathological conditions.

The Shorter the Vibrating Portion, the Smaller the Amplitude. Examples of physiological variations in length of the vibrating portion are children's vocal folds relative to adults' and females' relative to males.' A pathological cause of a shortening of the vibrating portion is laryngeal web.

The Stiffer the Vocal Fold Tissue, the Smaller the Amplitude. An example is phonation at high fundamental frequency, especially in falsetto voice, as a normal variation. Carcinoma, papilloma, scar, sulcus vocalis, firm nodule, and firm polyp are pathological examples.

The Greater the Mass of Vocal Fold, the Smaller the Amplitude. Examples are carcinoma, papilloma, polyp, and Reinke's edema.

The Existence of an Obstacle Decreases Amplitude. Examples are excessive masses such as carcinoma, papilloma, polyp, or cyst of the contralateral vocal fold.

The Greater the Subglottal Pressure, the Greater the Amplitude. An example is loud phonation.

Too Tight Glottal Closure Results in a Small Amplitude. Examples are spastic dysphonia and hyperkinetic phonation.

Glottal Closure

Judgment and Description

Glottal closure is rated overall as "complete" or "incomplete" and is determined by the extent of vocal fold approximation during the maximum closing of the vibratory cycle:

> *Complete.* The glottis is completely closed during each vibratory cycle.
>
> *Incomplete.* The glottis is never closed during the vibratory cycle.
>
> *Inconsistent.* The glottis is completely closed during some vibratory cycles, and incompletely closed during others.

When the glottis is completely closed, it is advisable to describe qualitatively the length of the closed phase as "very long," "long," "fairly long," "short," or "very short." When the glottal closure is incomplete, it is advisable to specify the shape of the glottis at the maximum closing (Figure 5–3).

Interpretation

An incomplete glottal closure during vocal fold vibration can result from a number of conditions.

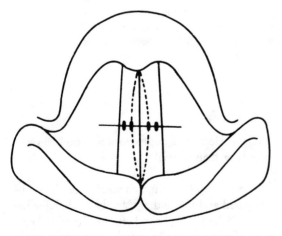

Figure 5–2. Schematic illustrates amplitude changes of the vocal folds. The center line is no visible movement, the first mark normal, and the second illustrates great movement.

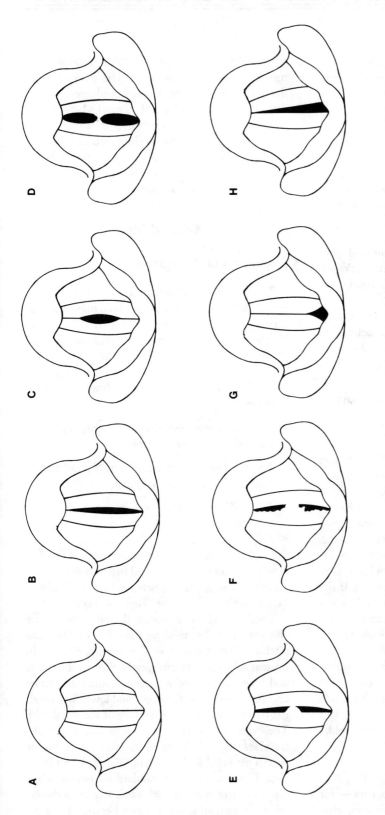

Figure 5–3. Sketches represent typical glottal closure patterns. (A) Complete closure; (B) Spindle-shaped gap along the entire length; (C) Spindle-shaped gap at middle; (D) Hourglass-shaped gap; (E) Gap by unilateral oval mass; (F) Gap with irregular shape; (G) Gap at posterior glottis; and (H) Gap along entire length.

Impaired Adduction of Vocal Fold(s). Impaired adduction can be caused by recurrent laryngeal nerve paralysis, ankylosis, or luxation of the cricoarytenoid joint(s).

Nonlinear Edge. Nonlinearity can be caused by a nodule, polyp, cyst, papilloma, or carcinoma.

Obstacle Between the Vocal Folds. Intervening obstacles could be a foreign body, a web, or a granuloma.

Stiff Edge. If the edge is stiff, no mucosal wave occurs or the Bernoulli effect does not work efficiently. Causes can be a scar or sulcus vocalis.

Dominant Cricothyroid Activity. If cricothyroid activity overpowers the adductor muscles, as in the production of a falsetto voice, glottal closure is compromised.

Symmetry of Bilateral Movement

Judgment and Description

Symmetry is based on the degree to which the two vocal folds provide mirror images of one another during vibration. The symmetry of the timing of opening, closing, and closure, and extent of lateromedial excursion of the folds are described in two ways (Figure 5–4). If the timing of opening, closing, and closure and the extent of latero-medial excursion during vibration appear the same for both vocal folds, movement is regarded as symmetrical. If the timing of opening, closing, and closure and/or extent of lateral excursion during vibration do not appear to be the same for both vocal folds, movement is considered to be asymmetrical.

If the movements of the vocal folds are asymmetrical, it is advisable to describe the asymmetry — for example, "The amplitude is greater on the right side than on the left," or "The excursion of the right vocal fold lags behind that of the left vocal fold."

Interpretation

Any differences in mechanical properties — for example, the position, shape, mass, tension, elasticity, and viscosity of the vocal folds — cause asymmetrical vibratory movements. The examiner who finds asymmetrical vibration should speculate on differences in the mechanical properties between the two vocal folds even though they look quite alike.

Any unilateral lesion provides an example of these differences. Differences in motor control between the two folds might also be associated with neurological or functional diseases.

Mucosal Wave

Judgment and Description

The occurrence of mucosal waves traveling the vertical length of the vocal folds is an important feature of vibration. The waves are not fixed, but rather identifiable in a specific phase of vibration. Mucosal waves can be described in four ways.

Absent. No observable traveling wave is present.

Small. The traveling wave is present, but less marked than normal range.

Normal. There is a clearly observable traveling mucosal wave of normal range.

Great. The traveling wave is extraordinarily marked.

In addition, the relative displacement of the mucosal wave should be compared between the two vocal folds. The results are then described as "Right > Left," "Right = Left," or "Right < Left."

The "normal range" means the range of the size and extent of the traveling wave for the "habitual pitch and habitual loudness" in normal subjects. In normal subjects, one can clearly observe the upper and lower lips at and after the maximum opening and also one can see the upper and lower lips traveling laterally on the upper surface of the vocal fold. The extent this wave travels varies, but it normally traverses at least half the entire width of the visible part of the vocal fold during normal pitch and loudness. This can serve as a standard for normal when one evaluates the mucosal wave. Children display relatively marked mucosal waves because they have

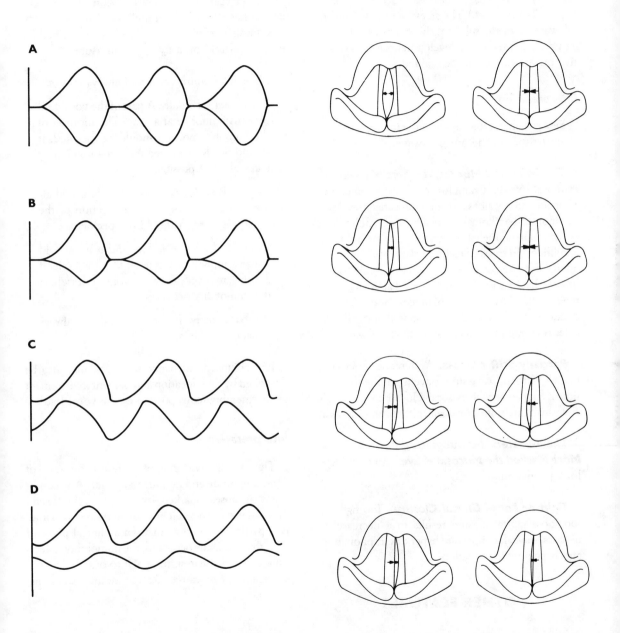

Figure 5–4. Glottal waveforms depict symmetrical and asymmetrical vibration. In each tracing, the top waveform represents movement of the left vocal fold and the bottom waveform represents movement of the right vocal fold. (A) Movement is symmetrical; (B) Movement is asym- metrical in amplitude with the right fold moving less than the left; (C) Movement is asymmetrical in phase but amplitudes are similar; and (D) Movement is asymmetrical in both amplitude and phase.

relatively thick pliable mucosa. (See Chapter 2, Figures 2–3 and 2–4.) The assessment of the mucosal wave is made subjectively at present. It, too, awaits further technical developments before objective quantification can be realized.

Interpretation

Several general rules apply in the interpretation of characteristics of the mucosal wave.

The Stiffer the Mucosa, the Less Marked the Mucosal Wave. Examples are a falsetto voice and phonation in dry air as physiological variations. Scars, carcinomas, papillomas, cysts, fibrotic nodules, firm polyps, and epithelial hyperplasia are pathological conditions. In cases of recurrent laryngeal nerve paralysis, the mucosa is stiffened because the vocalis muscle that opposes the cricothyroid activity is inactive, resulting in a decrease of mucosal wave. In cases of edematous lesions, the mucosa is abnormally pliable, resulting in an increase in mucosal wave.

Partially Stiff Mucosa. When the mucosa is partially stiff, the wave stops traveling at the stiff portion. Examples are sulcus vocalis, localized scar, small cyst, small carcinoma, or small epithelial hyperplasia.

The Greater the Subglottal Pressure, the More Marked the Mucosal Wave. An example is loud phonation.

Tight or Loose Glottal Closure. Too tight or too loose glottal closure results in a decrease of mucosal wave. Examples are hyperkinetic phonation and hypokinetic phonation.

OTHER FEATURES

Nonvibrating Portions

Judgment and Description

If any portion of the vocal fold does not vibrate — in other words, remains immobile during phonation — this should be specified. The absence of vibratory movement can occur either occasionally or always, and either partially or entirely on the vocal folds. The findings of immobility should be described for each vocal fold on a five-point measure.

None. The entire vocal fold always moves.

Occasionally, Partially. A part of the vocal fold remains immobile at a time. The location of the immobile portion should be specified. It should be also specified *when* the immobility takes place, if possible.

Always, Partially. A part of the vocal fold always remains immobile. The location of the immobile portion should be specified.

Occasionally, Entirely. The entire vocal fold remains immobile at a time. It is advisable, if possible, to specify the conditions under which the immobility occurs.

Always, Entirely. The entire vocal fold always remains immobile.

Immobility, or adynamic segments, may also be described by their location and percent involvement of the membraneous portion of the vocal folds.

Interpretation

The immobility during phonation is the state of "zero amplitude and no mucosal wave." Any condition that causes a marked decrease in amplitude and mucosal wave can result in a nonvibrating vocal fold. It is particularly important from a clinical point of view that, on many occasions, the immobility reflects a marked increase in stiffness of the vocal fold mucosa. Examples of causes are carcinoma, papilloma, or scar.

Other Findings at the Glottis

If any other findings are made, it is advisable to describe them. Examples of such occurrences are:

- A polyp moves with a delay from the vocal fold proper;

- The edge of the right vocal fold crosses the midline toward the end of the medial excursion to reach the left vocal fold;
- The edge of the left vocal fold crosses the midline toward the end of the medial excursion but does not reach the right vocal fold; or
- The bilateral vocal processes of the arytenoid cartilages are involved in vibratory movements.

Supraglottal Observations

In normal conditions, the supraglottic structures are not involved in vibratory movements. They remain stationary. In some pathological states, however, part(s) of the supraglottic structures might vibrate. If this is the case, it should be described.

Examples of supraglottal phenomena are:

- The bilateral false folds are vibrating;
- The left arytenoid region displays vibration;
- The right arytenoid region and the base of the epiglottis present with irregular vibration;
- The entire glottal structure is seen to tremor; or
- The supraglottal structures squeeze together.

Vibrations of the supraglottal structures take place when the vocal fold(s) is (are) severely damaged. This is a compensatory mechanism and seen sometimes after hemilaryngectomy and in cases of post-traumatic scarring.

This brief set of guidelines prepares the clinician for the initial assessment of laryngeal pathology. These clinical implications are the next step in understanding and treating a laryngeal condition.

STUDY QUESTIONS

1. The following parameters of vocal fold vibration should be described by the examiner:

   a. Fundamental frequency and periodicity.

   b. Horizontal and vertical movements.

   c. Mucosal wave.

   d. Opening and closing phases.

   e. All of the above.

2. Changes in fundamental frequency can be described as follows:

   a. The stiffer the vocal fold tissue, the smaller the mucosal wave.

   b. The shorter the vibrating portion of the vocal fold, the greater the fundamental frequency.

   c. The greater the mass of the vocal fold, the smaller the fundamental frequency.

   d. None of the above.

3. Periodicity describes:

   a. Open and closed phases.

   b. Regularity of successive movements.

   c. Superior/inferior movements of the wave.

   d. Activity of the vocal folds during a period of rest.

4. The scale used to rate amplitude includes the following intervals:

   a. Zero, small, average, great.

   b. Zero, small, normal, large.

   c. Zero, small, normal, great.

   d. None, small, great.

5. Glottic closure can be described as:

   a. None or all.

   b. Complete, incomplete, or inconsistent.

   c. Maximum, minimum, or normal.

   d. None of the above.

6. Mucosal wave describes waves traveling:

   a. The vertical length of the vocal fold.

b. Horizontally on the vocal fold.

c. Mucosal wave is not an important feature of vibration.

7. Supraglottic activity:

a. Is not related to vibratory activity of the vocal folds.

b. Is important in identifying some pathological states.

c. Is sometimes a compensatory mechanism.

d. b and c.

e. a and c.

CHAPTER

6

Typical Vibratory Patterns in Vocal Pathologies and Their Clinical Implications

No specific disease or pathology of the phonatory system always displays a given vibratory pattern. The vibratory pattern depends not only on the disease itself, but also on the size, degree, extent, and histological pattern of the disease and the manner of phonation, including compensatory behavior. There is no consistent relationship between a disease and a vibratory pattern. There are, however, general vibratory tendencies resulting from the deviation in mechanical properties of the vocal fold tissue caused by a given disease. Thus, a typical vibratory pattern of the vocal fold can frequently be associated with specific diseases.

We describe here the vibratory pattern of the vocal fold observed most commonly in 19 pathologies. They are presented in relation to the mechanical properties of the vocal fold and aerodynamic characteristics. In discussing the vocal fold as a vibrator in pathological states, 13 variables should be taken into consideration; these are presented in the figures that accompany each example.

ACUTE CATARRHAL LARYNGITIS

In acute catarrhal laryngitis (Figure 6–1), the pathology is located in the superficial layer of the lamina propria. If an edematous lesion is dominant, the cover becomes abnormally pliable. On the other hand, when infiltration of white blood cell and/or capillary dilation is dominant, the cover becomes stiff. The mass of the cover is slightly increased.

Abnormality in vibratory pattern is often minimal. A markedly edematous lesion might result in aperiodic vibrations. If there is a marked increase in stiffness, vibratory movements are highly limited, resulting in incomplete glottal closure and a very small amplitude of movement or — in rare instances — no observable vibration.

Acute Catarrhal Laryngitis (Unilateral)

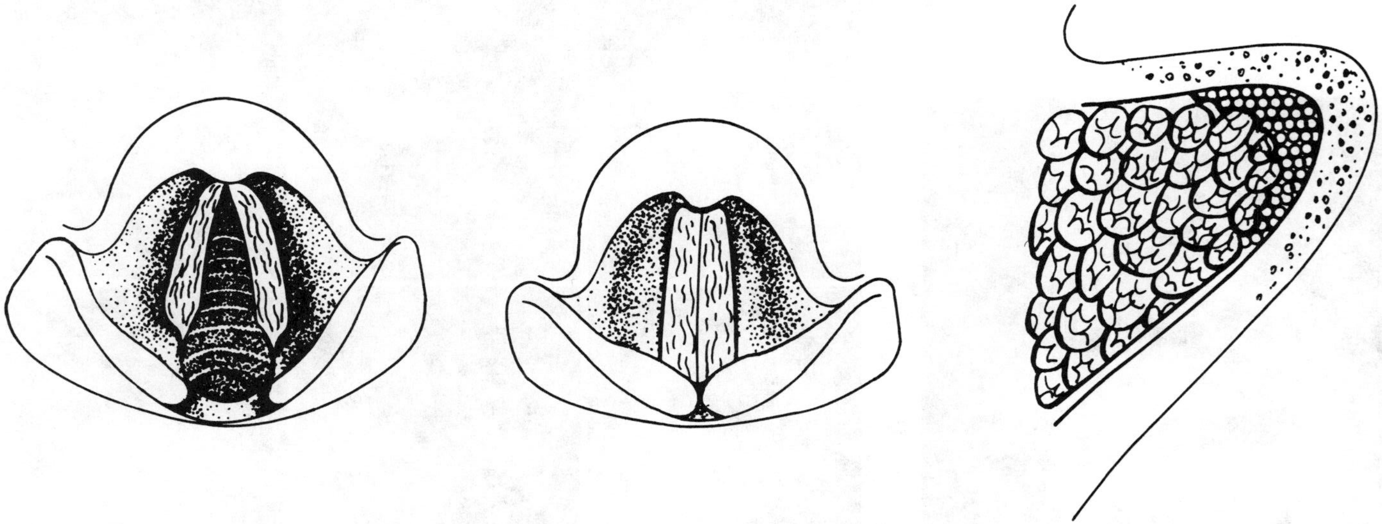

Location of pathology: *Superficial layer of lamina propria (cover)*

Glottal incompetence: None

Symmetry: Almost symmetrical

Homogeneity: Almost homogeneous

Edge: Almost linear

Length: Normal

Cover: Stiffness: *Varying*

       Mass: *Slightly increased*

Transition: Stiffness: Normal

            Mass: Normal

Body: Stiffness: Normal

      Mass: Normal

Obstacle: None

Tonus of adductor muscles: Consistent, almost normal

Expiratory force: Almost normal

Subglottal pressure: Almost normal

Figure 6–1. (A) Views of the larynx during respiration and phonation; a schematic of the vocal fold in a frontal section; and the mechanical and aero- dynamic aspects for acute catarrhal laryngitis. (B) Videostroboscopic prints of a case of acute catarrhal laryngitis.

A

Figure 6–1 *(continued)*

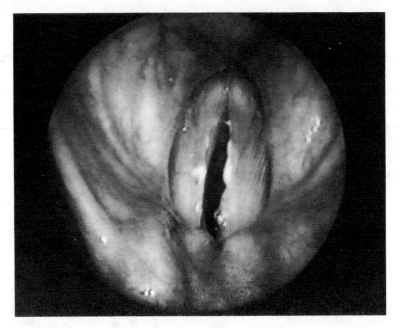

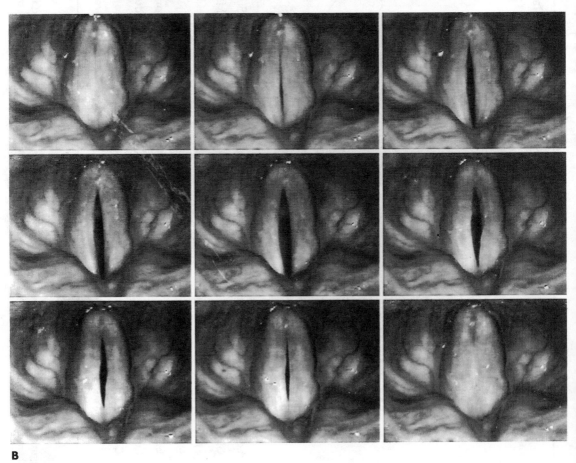

B

CHRONIC CATARRHAL LARYNGITIS

The pathology in chronic catarrhal laryngitis (Figure 6-2) is located in the superficial layer of the lamina propria and occasionally also in the epithelium. The stiffness of the cover is often increased because the lesion often consists of infiltration of lymphocytes and plasma cells, an increase in fibrous tissue, and thickening of the epithelium. If edema is the dominant feature, the stiffness might be reduced. The mass of the cover is slightly increased.

Abnormality in the vibratory pattern is frequently minimal. Both the amplitude and mucosal wave tend to be reduced.

Chronic Catarrhal Laryngitis (Bilateral)

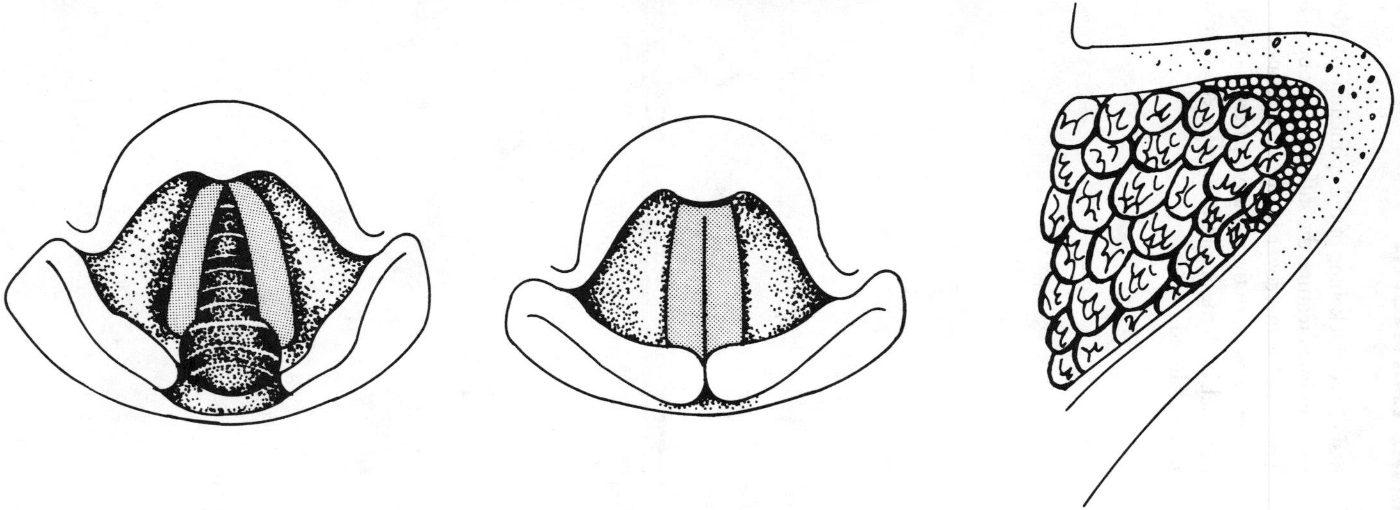

Location of pathology: *Superficial layer of lamina propria (cover)*

Glottal incompetence: None

Symmetry: Almost symmetrical

Homogeneity: Almost homogeneous

Edge: Almost linear

Length: Normal

Cover: Stiffness: *Varying (often increased)*

　　　Mass: *Slightly increased*

Transition: Stiffness: Normal

　　　　　　Mass: Normal

Body: Stiffness: Normal

　　　Mass: Normal

Obstacle: None

Tonus of adductor muscles: Consistent, almost normal

Expiratory force: Almost normal

Subglottal pressure: Almost normal

Figure 6–2. (A) Views of the larynx; a schematic of the vocal fold in a frontal section; and the mechanical and aerodynamic aspects for chronic catarrhal laryngitis. (B) Videostroboscopic prints of a case of chronic catarrhal laryngitis.

A

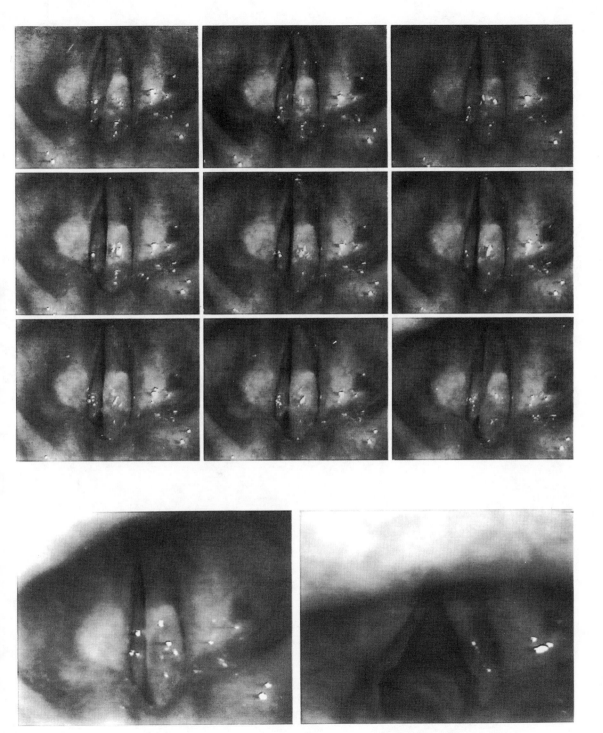

B

SUBEPITHELIAL BLEEDING OF THE VOCAL FOLD

Subepithelial bleeding takes place usually as an acute trauma caused by abusive phonation. The lesion is often unilateral (Figure 6–3).

The pathology is located in the superficial layer of the lamina propria. Because the lesion is often unilateral, the mechanical properties of the bilateral vocal folds are asymmetrical. On the affected side, the stiffness of the cover is increased and the mass of the cover is slightly increased. The amplitude and mucosal wave on the affected side are smaller than those on the unaffected side, resulting in asymmetrical vibratory movements. The asymmetry can be in both phase and amplitude.

Subepithelial Bleeding (Unilateral)

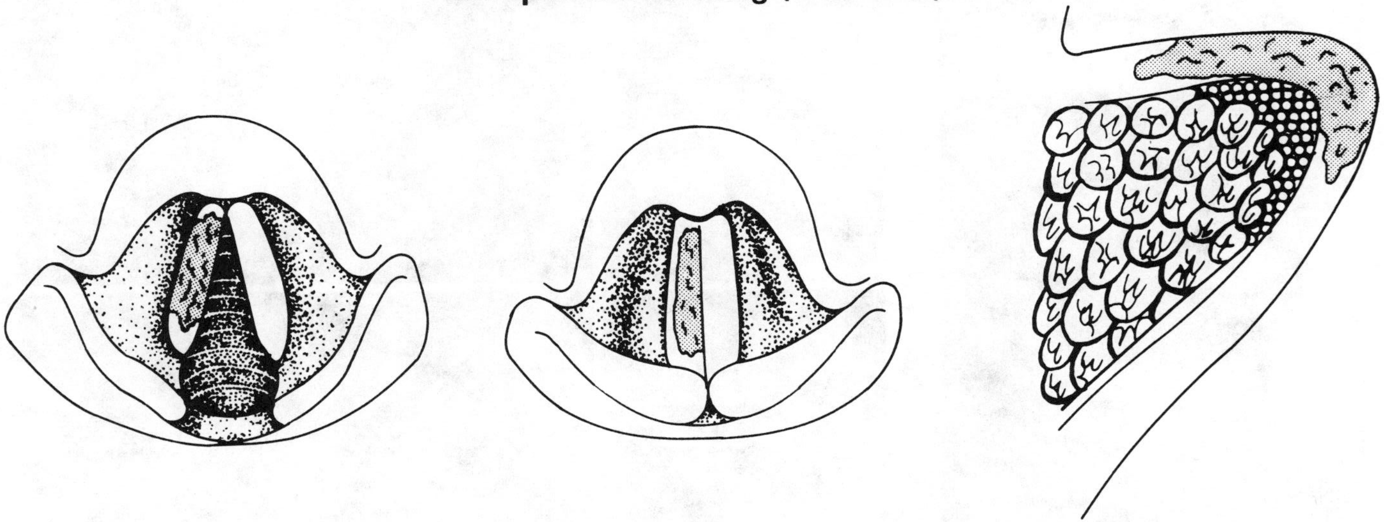

Location of pathology: *Superficial layer of lamina propria (cover)*

Glottal incompetence: None

Symmetry: Asymmetrical

Homogeneity: Almost homogeneous

Edge: Almost linear

Length: Normal

Cover: Stiffness: *Increased*

　　　Mass: *Slightly increased*

Transition: Stiffness: Normal

　　　Mass: Normal

Body: Stiffness: Normal

　　　Mass: Normal

Obstacle: None

Tonus of adductor muscles: Consistent, almost normal

Expiratory force: Almost normal

Subglottal pressure: Almost normal

A

Figure 6-3. (A) Views of the larynx; a schematic of the vocal fold in a frontal section; and the mechanical and aerodynamic aspects for subepithelial bleed-ing. (B) Videostroboscopic prints of a case of subepithelial bleeding.

Figure 6–3 *(continued)*

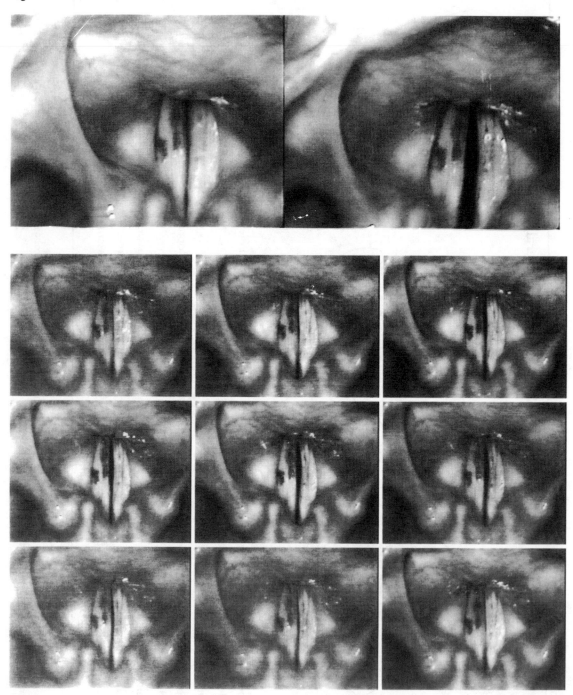

B

VOCAL FOLD NODULES

Vocal fold nodules (Figure 6–4) result from chronic abusive phonation. The lesion is usually bilateral.

The pathology is located in the superficial layer of the lamina propria. The glottis does not close anterior and posterior to the nodules. The lesion is usually nearly symmetrical. The structure of each vocal fold is slightly heterogeneous because of the existence of the nodule. The vocal fold edge is nonlinear because the nodule produces a small bump. The nature of the stiffness of the cover varies depending on the histological feature — that is, the stiffness is increased in fibrous nodules, whereas it is reduced in edematous nodules. The mass of the cover is slightly increased. The nodules interfere slightly with the vibratory movements of the contralateral vocal fold.

During vibration, the glottal closure is incomplete, presenting with an hourglass glottis at the maximum closure. The amplitude is usually reduced bilaterally. The mucosal wave is absent at the nodule when the nodule is fibrous and firm. If the nodule is edematous and soft, the mucosal wave is often observed on the nodule. By looking at the mucosal wave, therefore, one can estimate the histological characteristics of the nodule to a limited extent.

Vocal Fold Nodule (Bilateral)

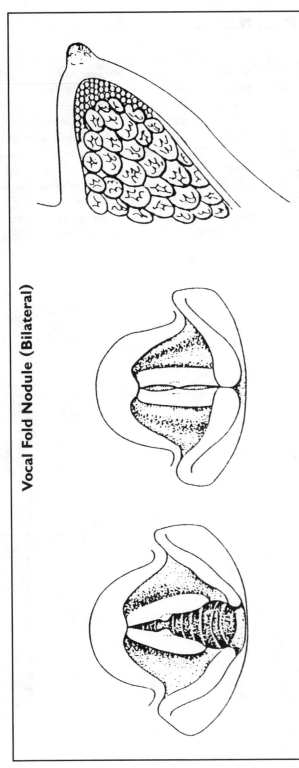

Location of pathology: *Superficial layer of lamina propria (cover)*

Glottal incompetence: *Partly*

Symmetry: Almost symmetrical

Homogeneity: *Heterogeneous*

Edge: *Nonlinear*

Length: Normal

Cover: Stiffness: *Varying*

       Mass: *Slightly increased*

Transition: Stiffness: Normal

          Mass: Normal

Body: Stiffness: Normal

     Mass: Normal

Obstacle: *Present*

Tonus of adductor muscles: Consistent, almost normal

Expiratory force: Almost normal

Subglottal pressure: Almost normal

A

Figure 6–4. (A) Views of the larynx; a schematic drawing of the vocal fold in a frontal section; and the mechanical and aerodynamic aspects of vocal fold nodules. (B) through (F) Videostroboscopic prints of a case of vocal fold nodules.

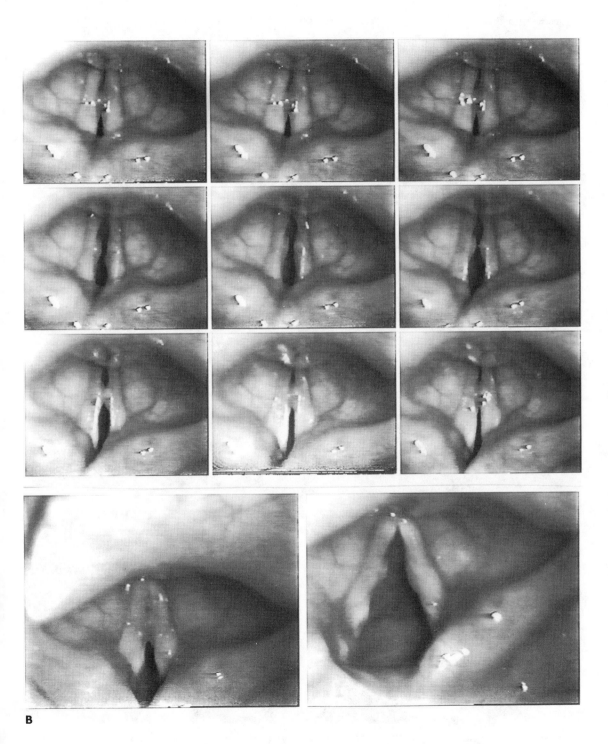

B

Figure 6–4 *(continued)*

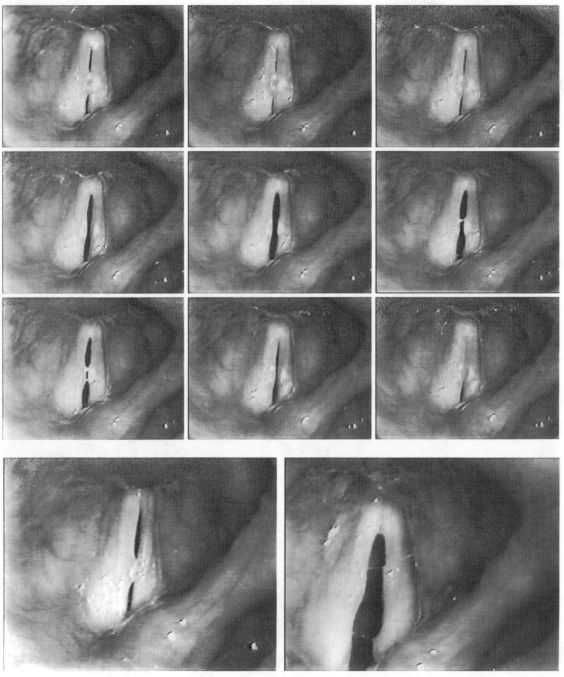

C

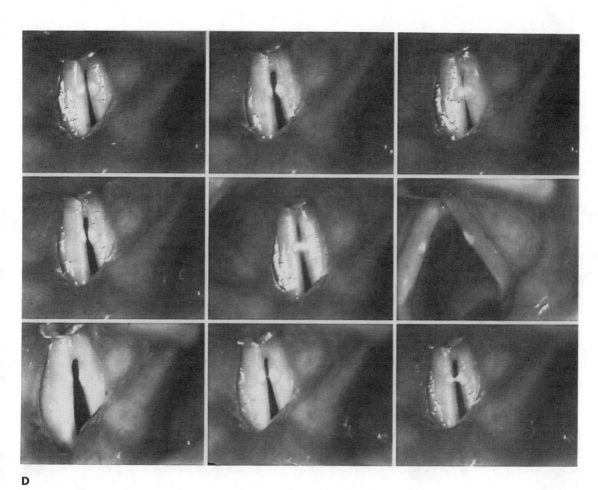

D

Figure 6–4 (continued)

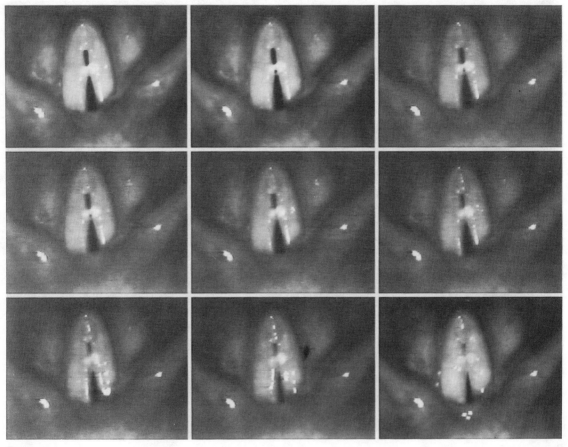

E

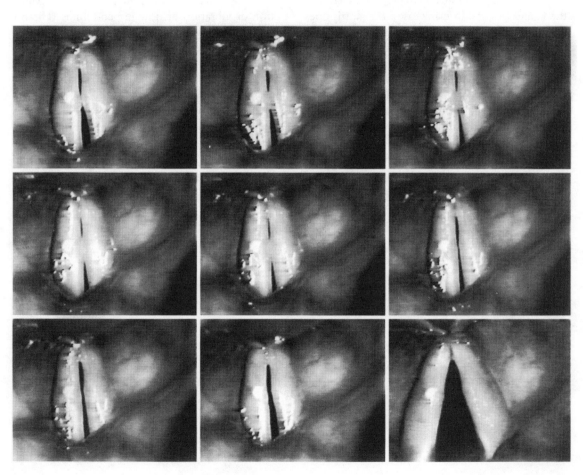

F

VOCAL FOLD POLYPS

Vocal fold polyps (Figure 6–5) can also result from abusive phonation, as well as a number of other factors. The lesion can be unilateral or bilateral, but a unilateral lesion is more frequent. When bilateral, the polyps are usually asymmetrical.

The pathology is located in the superficial layer of the lamina propria. In many cases, the glottis does not close anterior and posterior to the polyp. The bilateral vocal folds are asymmetrical and the affected vocal fold is heterogeneous in structure. The edge of the vocal fold is nonlinear as a result of the configuration created by the polyp. The stiffness of the cover varies: When the polyp is hemorrhagic or fibrous, the stiffness is increased; if the polyp is edematous, the stiffness is decreased. The mass of the cover is increased. The polyp can interfere with the vibratory movements of the contralateral vocal fold. Expiratory force and subglottal pressure are usually near normal. They are increased when phonation becomes strained.

During vibration, the glottal closure is incomplete, presenting with gaps anterior and posterior to the polyp during maximum closure. The vibratory movements of the vocal folds are usually asymmetrical. The polyps usually move with a slight lag behind the vocal fold proper, presenting with coupled vibration or vibration of double pendulums (Hirano, Matsushita, Kawasaki, Yoshida, & Koike, 1974). Successive vibrations are often aperiodic. The amplitude of the affected vocal fold is small and that of the contralateral vocal fold is often slightly reduced because of the interference caused by the polyp. The mucosal wave on the polyp is usually absent when the polyp is hemorrhagic or fibrous, but it is of normal size or greater if the polyp is edematous and pliable. One can, therefore, also speculate about the histological characteristics of polyps to some extent by means of stroboscopy.

Vocal Fold Polyp (Unilateral)

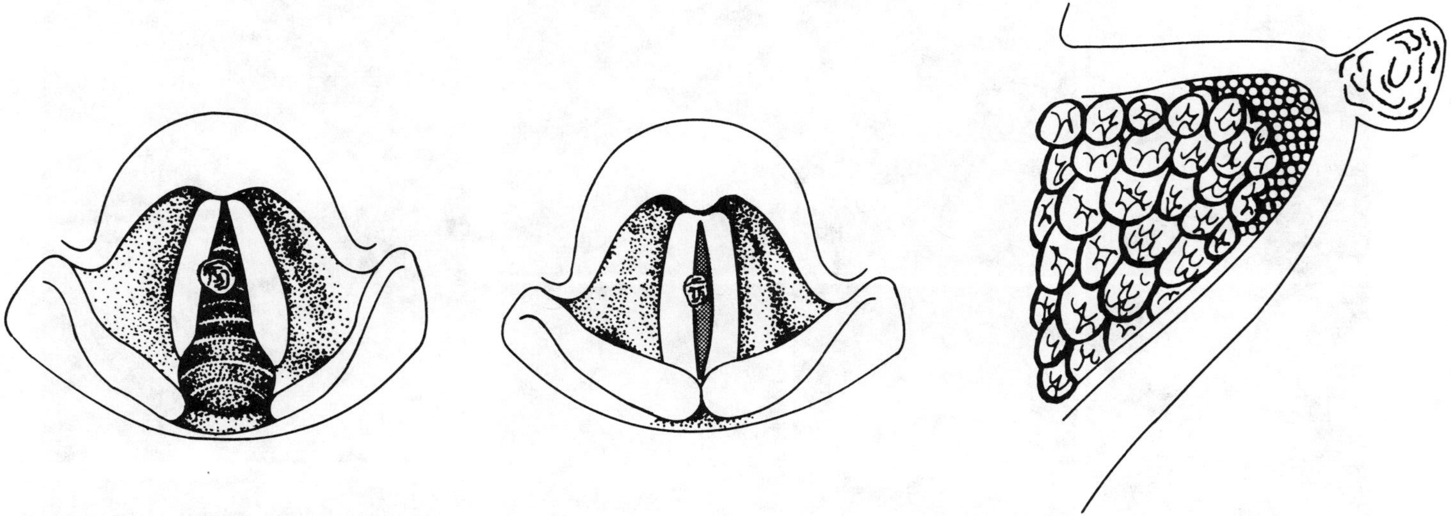

Location of pathology: *Superficial layer of lamina propria (cover)*

Glottal incompetence: *Partly*

Symmetry: *Asymmetrical*

Homogeneity: *Heterogeneous*

Edge: *Nonlinear*

Length: *Normal*

Cover: Stiffness: *Varying*

      Mass: Normal

Transition: Stiffness: Normal

         Mass: Normal

Body: Stiffness: Normal

      Mass: Normal

Obstacle: *Present*

Tonus of adductor muscles: Consistent, almost normal

Expiratory force: Almost normal, occasionally increased

Subglottal pressure: Almost normal, occasionally increased

Figure 6–5. (A) Views of the larynx; a schematic of the vocal fold in a frontal section; and the mechanical and aerodynamic aspects for a unilateral vocal fold polyp. (B) and (C) Videostroboscopic prints of a case of unilateral vocal fold polyp.

A

137

Figure 6–5 *(continued)*

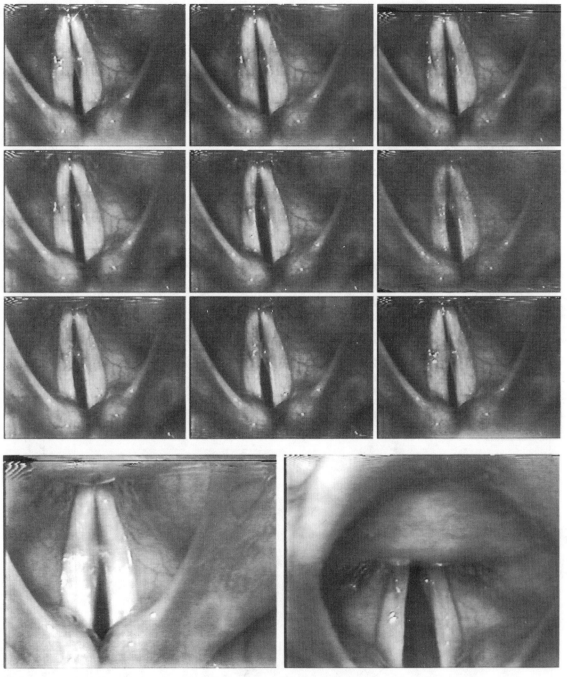

B

138

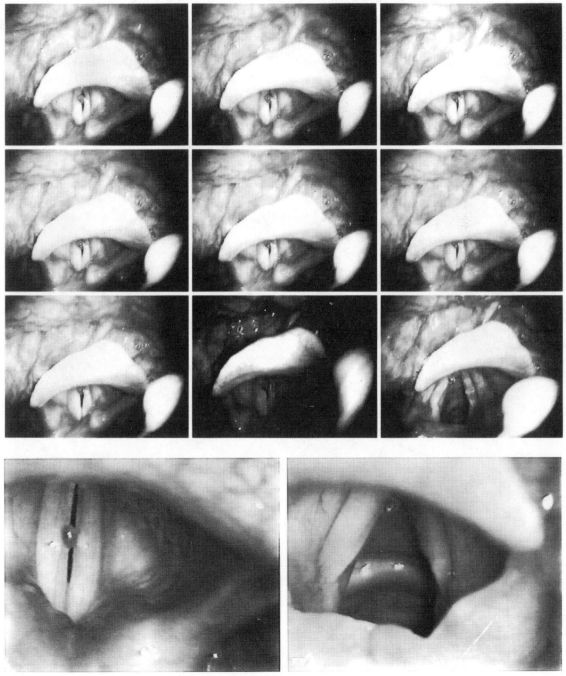

C

REINKE'S EDEMA
(Polypoid Degeneration, Polypoid Vocal Fold)

The etiology of this pathology is unknown, but it is usually developed in smokers of middle age and older. The lesion is usually bilateral but often asymmetrical (Figure 6–6).

The pathology is located in the superficial layer of the lamina propria, (Reinke's space). The stiffness of the cover is decreased, whereas the mass of the cover and depth of the vibratory edge are increased. The edematous swelling often interferes with the vibratory movement of the contralateral vocal fold.

Generally, during vibration, the glottis is closed completely. The movements of the bilateral vocal folds are asymmetrical, and successive vibrations are often aperiodic. The amplitude of horizontal excursion is often small, but the mucosal wave is usually markedly great.

Reinke's Edema (Bilateral)

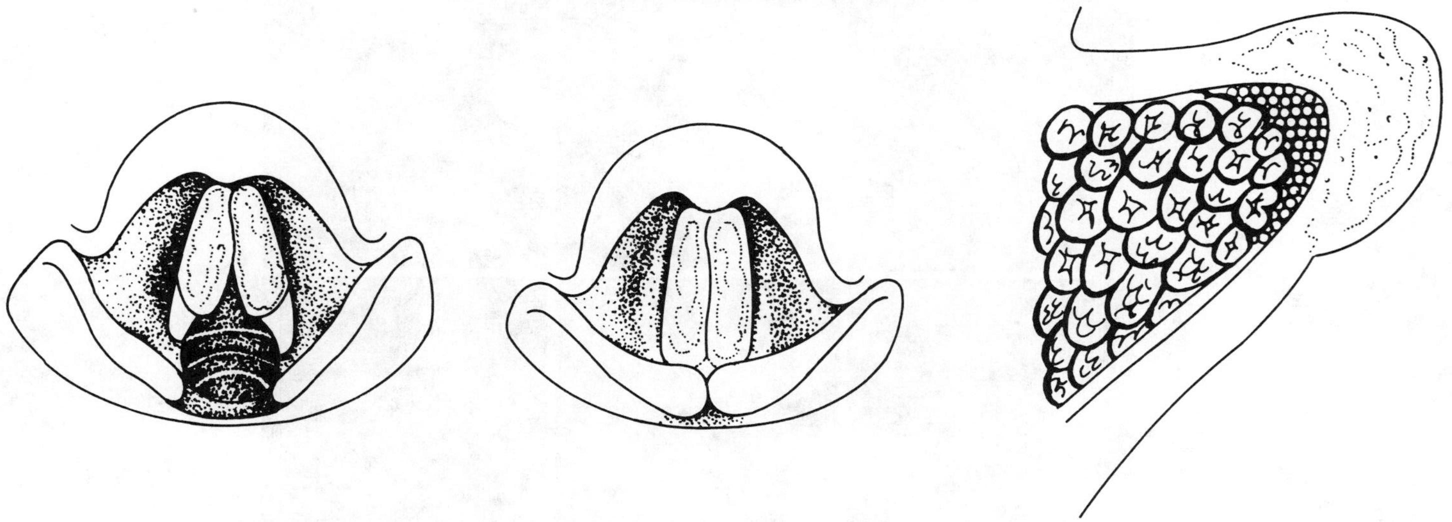

Location of pathology: *Superficial layer of lamina propria (cover)*

Glottal incompetence: None

Symmetry: *Asymmetrical*

Homogeneity: *Almost homogeneous*

Edge: Almost linear

Length: Normal

Cover: Stiffness: *Decreased*

Mass: *Increased*

Transition: Stiffness: Normal

Mass: Normal

Body: Stiffness: Normal

Mass: Normal

Obstacle: *Present*

Tonus of adductor muscles: Consistent, almost normal

Expiratory force: Almost normal

Subglottal pressure: Almost normal

Videostroboscopic prints of a case of Reinke's edema.

Figure 6-6. (A) Views of the larynx; a schematic of the vocal fold in frontal section; and the mechanical and aerodynamic aspects for Reinke's edema. (B)

A

Figure 6–6 (continued)

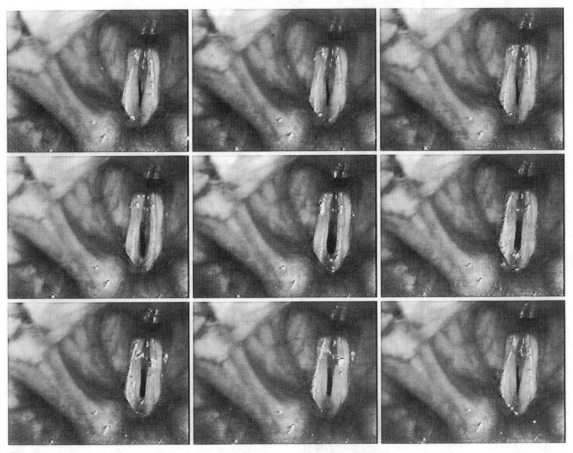

B

VOCAL FOLD CYSTS

Most cysts of the vocal fold are epidermoid cysts or retention cysts. They are almost always unilateral.

The pathology is located in the superficial layer of the lamina propria (Figure 6–7). The cyst is something like a small balloon full of fluid. The glottis often does not close anterior and posterior to the cyst. The mechanical properties are asymmetrical between the two vocal folds and heterogeneous within the affected vocal fold. The edge of the vocal fold is nonlinear because of the lump or protuberance caused by the cyst. The stiffness and mass of the cover is increased. Generally, cysts are stiffer than nodules and polyps. The cyst plays the role of being an obstacle against the contralateral vocal fold.

Glottal closure is often incomplete during vibration. Small gaps remain anterior and posterior to the cyst during maximum closure because the stiffness of the cyst when forced laterally by the impression of the two folds results in small chinks in the adjacent soft tissue. The vibratory movements of the two vocal folds are asymmetrical. Successive vibrations are sometimes aperiodic. The amplitude of lateral excursion is very small on the affected side and no mucosal wave is observed on the cyst. Cysts are usually differentiated from nodules and polyps by means of stroboscopic observation, for the limitations of vibration are much greater for cysts than for nodules and polyps.

Vocal Fold Cyst (Unilateral)

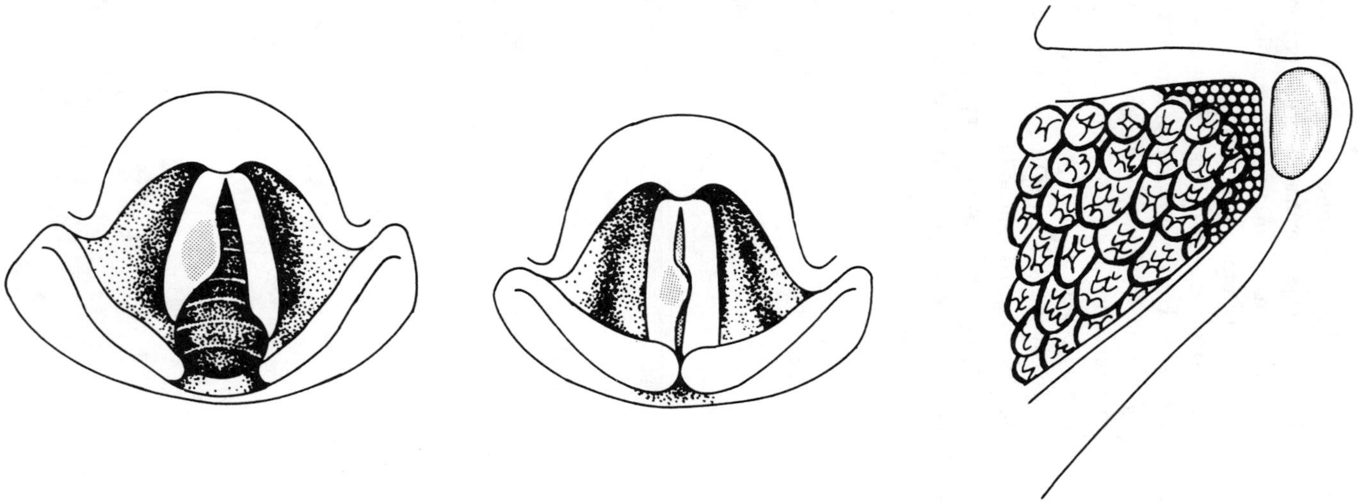

Location of pathology: *Superficial layer of lamina propria (cover)*

Glottal incompetence: *Partly*

Symmetry: *Asymmetrical*

Homogeneity: *Heterogeneous*

Edge: *Nonlinear*

Length: Normal

Cover: Stiffness: *Increased*

Mass: *Increased*

Transition: Stiffness: Normal

Mass: Normal

Body: Stiffness: Normal

Mass: Normal

Obstacle: *Present*

Tonus of adductor muscles: Consistent, almost normal

Expiratory force: Almost normal

Subglottal pressure: Almost normal

Videostroboscopic prints of a case of a vocal fold cyst.

A

Figure 6–7. (A) Views of the larynx; a schematic of the vocal fold in a frontal section; and the mechanical and aerodynamic aspects of vocal fold cysts. (B)

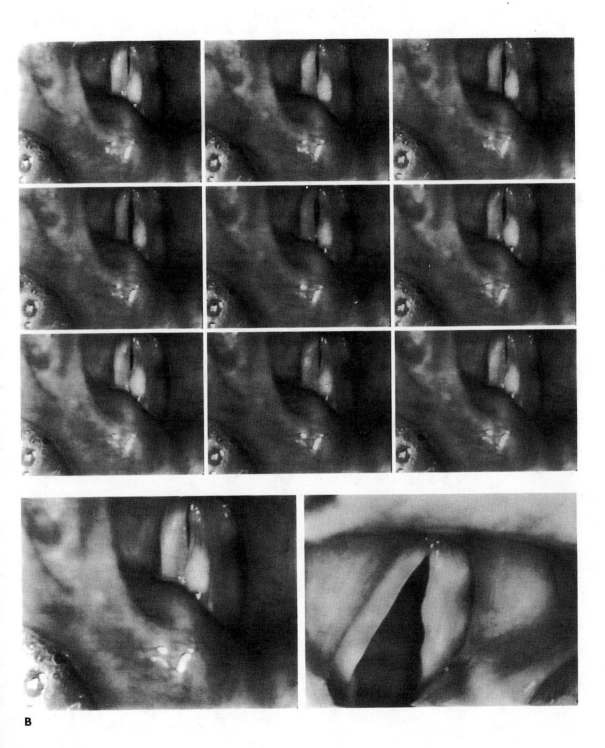

B

SULCUS VOCALIS

The term "sulcus vocalis" implies a condition in which a furrow along the edge of the vocal fold(s) causes voice disorders. The etiology of this disease is unknown but it is thought to be congenital in some cases and secondary to long-lasting or repeated chronic inflammatory processes in others. The lesion is usually bilateral and the furrow is located at the edge of the membranous vocal fold usually traversing the entire length of the membranous fold.

The lesion is located in the superficial layer of the lamina propria (Figure 6–8). The glottis is incompe-tent along the entire length, presenting a narrow spindle-shaped chink during phonation because the edges of the vocal folds are bowed. The stiffness of the cover is increased at the sulcus and the mass of the cover is slightly decreased.

During vibratory cycles, the glottal closure is incomplete. A thin, spindle-shaped gap remains in the glottis at the maximum closure. The amplitude of horizontal excursion is often reduced. The mucosal wave is interrupted at the furrow.

Sulcus Vocalis

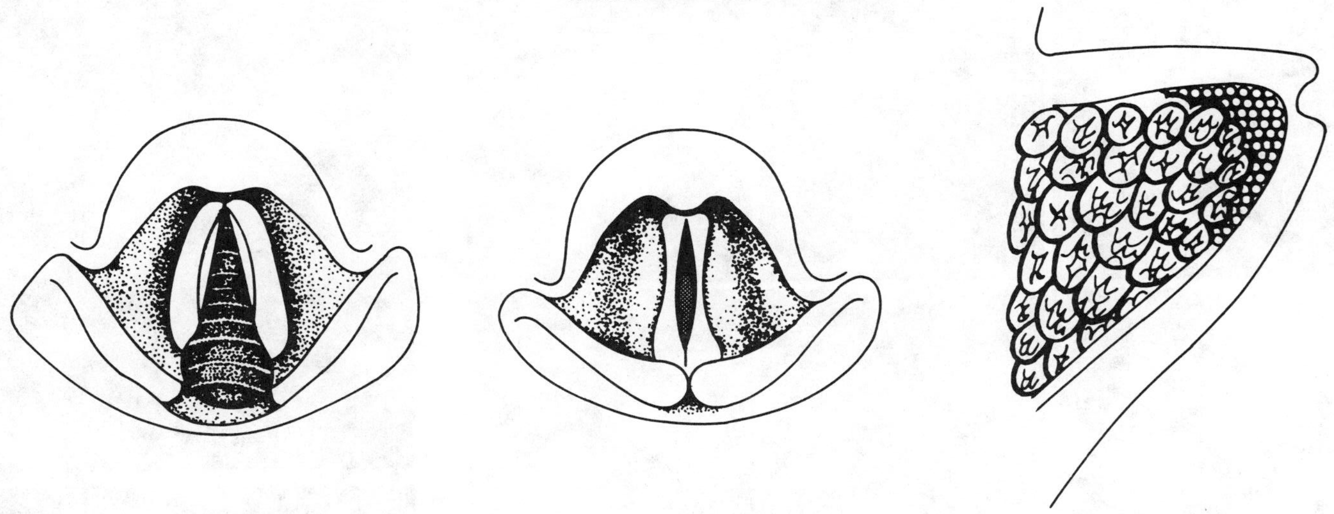

Location of pathology: *Superficial layer of lamina propria (cover)*

Glottal incompetence: *Along entire length,* slight

Symmetry: Almost symmetrical

Homogeneity: Almost homogeneous

Edge: *Bowed*

Length: Normal

Cover: Stiffness: *Increased*

    Mass: *Decreased*

Transition: Stiffness: Normal

    Mass: Normal

Body: Stiffness: Normal

    Mass: Normal

Obstacle: None

Tonus of adductor muscles: Consistent, almost normal

Expiratory force: Almost normal

Subglottal pressure: Almost normal

Figure 6–8. (A) Views of the larynx; a schematic of the vocal fold in a frontal section; and the mechanical and aerodynamic aspects for a sulcus vocalis. (B) Videostroboscopic prints of a case of sulcus vocalis.

A

147

Figure 6–8 (continued)

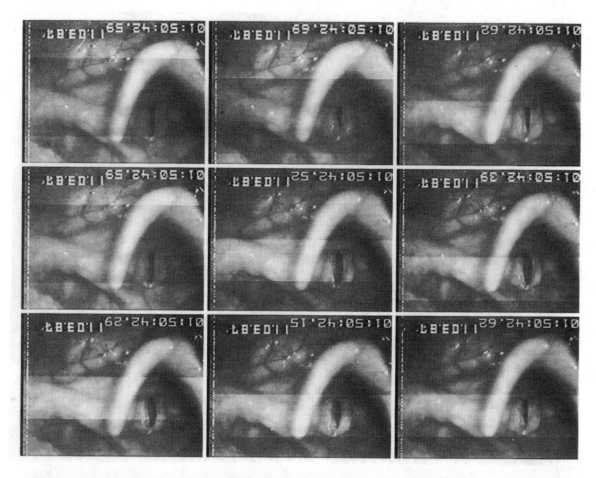

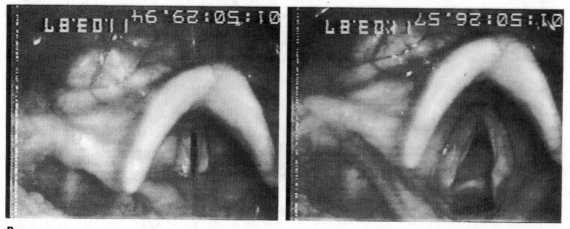

B

VOCAL FOLD SCARRING

Scar formation of the vocal fold usually results from trauma, including surgeries of the vocal fold. Occasionally it can be caused by inflammation. A small scar is often overlooked under traditional laryngeal examinations because its effect cannot be appreciated by the naked eye under standard light. The lesion can be either unilateral or bilateral.

The locations of the scar can vary. In this example (Figure 6–9), the glottal incompetence is slight. The mechanical properties of the bilateral vocal folds are usually asymmetrical. The affected vocal fold is homogeneous when the scar extends along the entire length. If the scar is localized, the vocal fold becomes heterogeneous in its mechanical properties. The stiff-

ness of the affected portion of the cover is always increased. When that happens, both the transitional layer and the body become stiff. The expiratory force and subglottal pressure often increase to force or blow the stiff structures apart and into vibration.

During the vibratory cycle, the glottis often does not close completely. The vibratory movements are asymmetrical between the two vocal folds and successive vibrations are frequently aperiodic. The amplitude of lateral excursions is reduced and little or no mucosal wave is observed in the cicatrice region. A small scar can be often detected only by a stroboscopic examination.

Vocal Fold Scarring

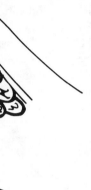

Location of pathology: *Varying*

Glottal incompetence: *In varying degrees*

Symmetry: *Asymmetrical*

Homogeneity: *Varying*

Edge: Usually linear

Length: Normal

Cover: Stiffness: *Increased*

Mass: *Varying*

Transition: Stiffness: Normal or *increased*

Mass: *Varying*

Body: Stiffness: Normal or *increased*

Mass: *Varying*

Obstacle: None

Tonus of adductor muscles: Consistent at varying level

Expiratory force: Presumably often *increased*

Subglottal pressure: Presumably often *increased*

Figure 6–9. (A) Views of the larynx; a schematic of a frontal section of the vocal fold; and the mechanical and aerodynamic aspects for a scar on a vocal fold. (B) Videostroboscopic prints of a case of vocal fold scarring.

A

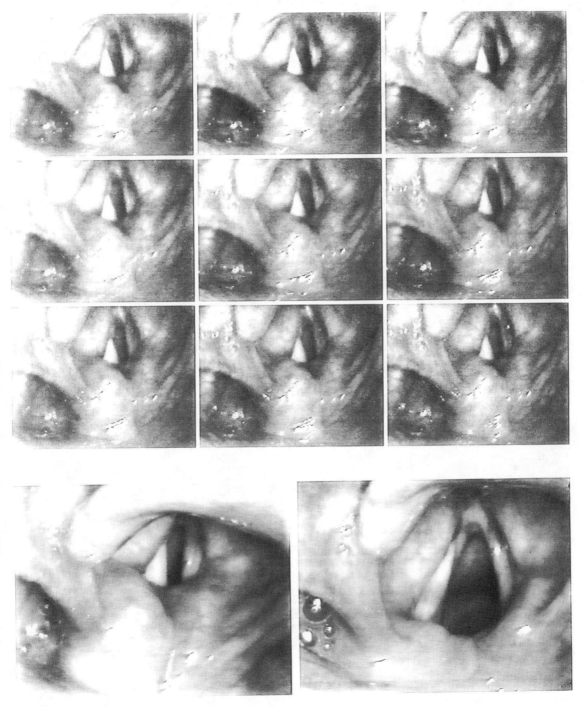

B

LARYNGEAL WEB

Laryngeal web is either congenital or acquired. It is usually developed at the anterior commissure (Figure 6–10).

The lesion is usually located at the anterior part of the glottis. During phonation, the glottis is closed or is open at a small area immediately posterior to the web. The length of the vibrating segment is shortened because of the existence of the web, which restricts motion to the portion of the vocal fold posterior to the web. This web, especially when it is thick and firm, can significantly interfere with vibratory movements of both vocal folds.

The fundamental frequency of phonation is usually high because the vibrating portion of the vocal fold is shortened. Similarly, for the same reason, the amplitude of horizontal excursion is small.

Laryngeal Web

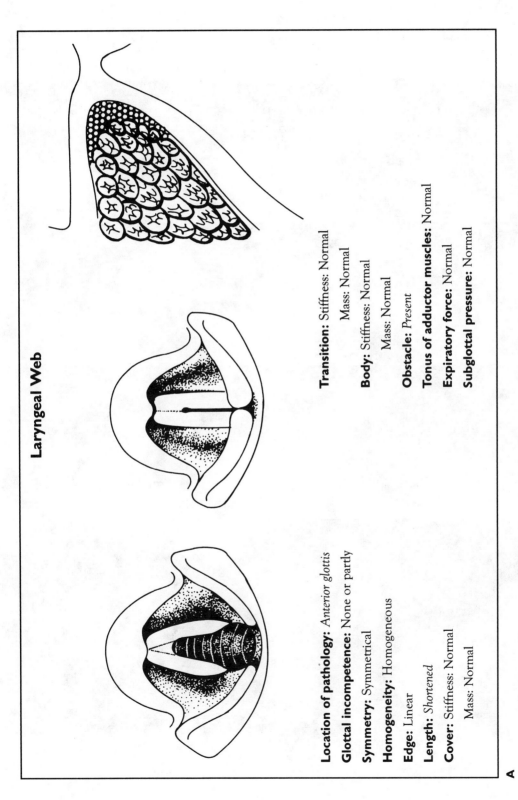

Location of pathology: *Anterior glottis*

Glottal incompetence: None or partly

Symmetry: Symmetrical

Homogeneity: Homogeneous

Edge: Linear

Length: *Shortened*

Cover: Stiffness: Normal

Mass: Normal

Transition: Stiffness: Normal

Mass: Normal

Body: Stiffness: Normal

Mass: Normal

Obstacle: *Present*

Tonus of adductor muscles: Normal

Expiratory force: Normal

Subglottal pressure: Normal

A

Figure 6–10. (A) Views of the larynx; a schematic of a frontal section of the vocal fold; and mechanical and aerodynamic aspects for laryngeal web. (B) Videostroboscopic prints of a case of laryngeal web.

Figure 6-10 *(continued)*

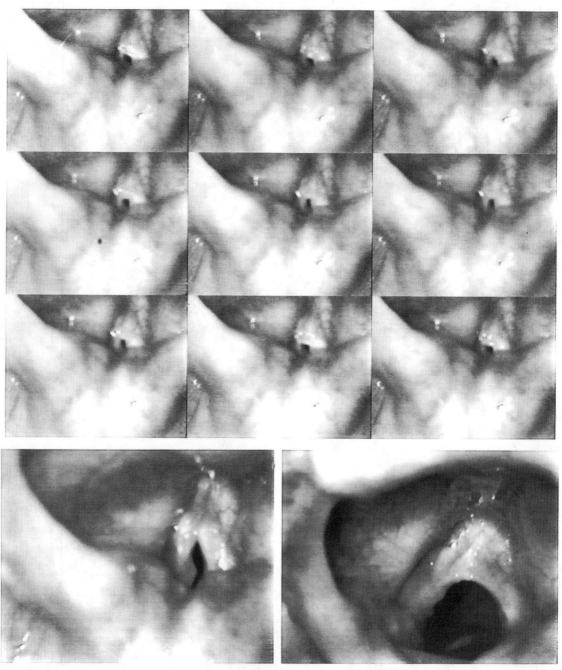

B

EPITHELIAL HYPERPLASIA/DYSPLASIA OF THE VOCAL FOLD

Epithelial hyperplasia has been referred to as leukoplakia, hyperkeratosis, keratosis, and acanthosis. The lesion can be unilateral or bilateral, exophytic, or plaque-like (Figure 6–11). Occasionally, it becomes malignant.

The lesion originates from the epithelium and enters the superficial layer of the lamina propria. It never invades the vocal ligament unless it becomes malignant. In many cases the glottis does not close completely. The mechanical properties of the two vocal folds are usually asymmetrical, even in the cases of bilateral involvement. The structure of the affected vocal fold(s) is heterogeneous. The edge of the vocal fold is often nonlinear. The stiffness and mass of the cover are increased. Expiratory force and subglottal pressure are usually near normal. They might be increased when the lesion is large.

During vibratory cycles, the glottal closure is often incomplete. A glottal chink of an irregular shape might involve a part or the entire length of the glottis. Vibratory movements of the two vocal folds are asymmetrical. Successive vibrations are often aperiodic. The amplitude of lateral excursion is limited. Occasionally, the lesion shows no movement when it is very thick. Mucosal wave is not observed at the site of the lesion. The limitation of vibratory movements is less in epithelial hyperplasia and dysplasia than in a carcinoma, which is associated with a deeper invasion of the underlying structure.

Epithelial Hyperplasia/Dysplasia (Leukoplakia) (Unilateral)

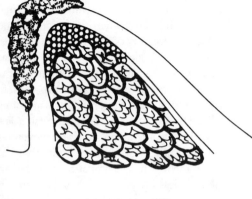

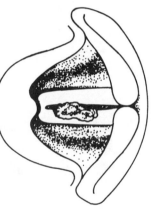

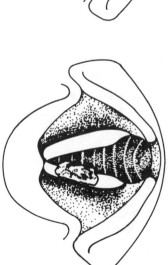

Location of pathology: Epithelium ⟶ *Superficial layer of lamina propria (cover)*

Glottal incompetence: *Occasionally partly or entirely*

Symmetry: *Asymmetrical*

Homogeneity: *Heterogeneous*

Edge: *Often nonlinear*

Length: Normal

Cover: Stiffness: *Increased*

　　　Mass: *Increased*

Transition: Stiffness: Normal

　　　　　　Mass: Normal

Body: Stiffness: Normal

　　　Mass: Normal

Obstacle: None

Tonus of adductor muscles: Consistent, almost normal

Expiratory force: Almost normal. Occasionally increased

Subglottal pressure: Almost normal. Occasionally increased

A

Figure 6–11. (A) Views of the larynx; a schematic of the vocal fold in a frontal section; and the mechanical and aerodynamic aspects of epithelial hyperplasia/ dysplasia. (B) Videostroboscopic prints of a case of hyperplasia/dysplasia.

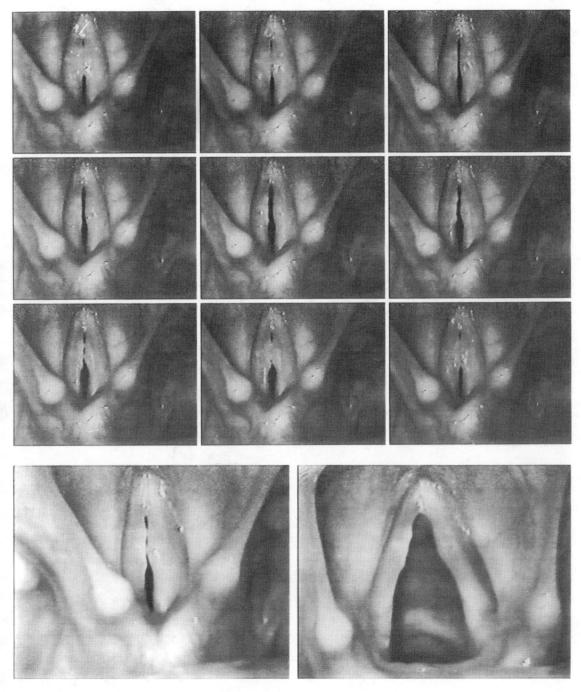

B

PAPILLOMA OF THE VOCAL FOLD

Papilloma of the larynx (Figure 6–12) is a benign neoplasm that is viral in origin. The lesion may be solitary or multiple.

The lesion originates from the epithelium but it can invade both the lamina propria of the mucosa and the muscle. The glottis is partly open because the edge(s) of the affected vocal fold(s) is (are) irregular and nonlinear. The bilateral vocal folds are asymmetrical even in the cases of bilateral lesions. The structure of the affected vocal fold is heterogeneous. The stiffness and mass of the cover are often markedly increased, as are those of the transition and body when the structures are invaded by papilloma. The extrusive papillomatous lesion interferes with the vibratory movements of the contralateral vocal fold in the speaker's effort to compensate for the stiff structures. The tonus of the adductor muscle is presumably increased, as are the expiratory force and subglottal pressure.

The glottis does not close completely during vibratory cycles, but shows a gap of irregular shape at the maximum closure. The vibratory movements of the two vocal folds are asymmetrical and successive vibrations are aperiodic. The amplitude of horizontal excursion is usually zero. In other words, the lesion is always nonvibrating and there is no mucosal wave on the papillomatous lesion.

Papilloma of the Vocal Fold (Unilateral)

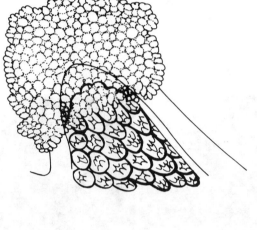

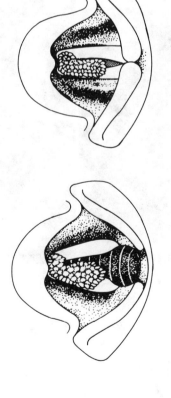

Location of pathology: *Epithelium* ⟶ *Lamina propria* ⟶ *Muscle (cover* ⟶ *body)*

Glottal incompetence: *Partly*

Symmetry: *Asymmetrical*

Homogeneity: *Heterogeneous*

Edge: *Nonlinear*

Length: *Normal*

Cover: Stiffness: *Increased* (markedly)

Mass: *Increased* (often markedly)

Transition: Stiffness: *Occasionally increased*

Mass: *Occasionally increased*

Body: Stiffness: *Occasionally increased*

Mass: *Occasionally increased*

Obstacle: *Present*

Tonus of adductor muscles: *Presumably often increased*

Expiratory force: *Presumably often increased*

Subglottal pressure: *Presumably often increased*

A

Figure 6–12. (A) Views of the larynx; a schematic of a frontal section of the vocal fold; and mechanical and aerodynamic aspects of papilloma of the vocal fold. (B) and (C) Videostroboscopic prints of a case of papilloma of the vocal fold.

Figure 6–12 *(continued)*

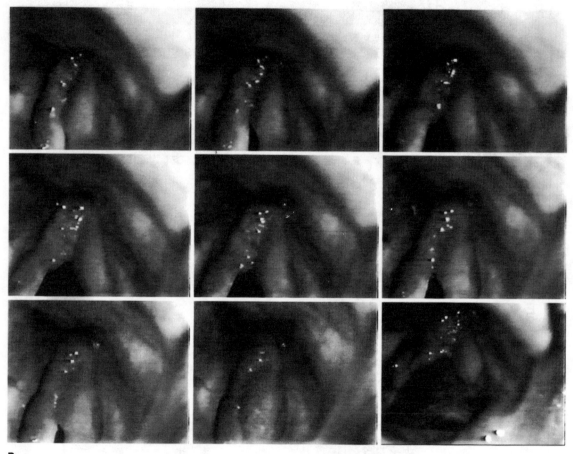

B

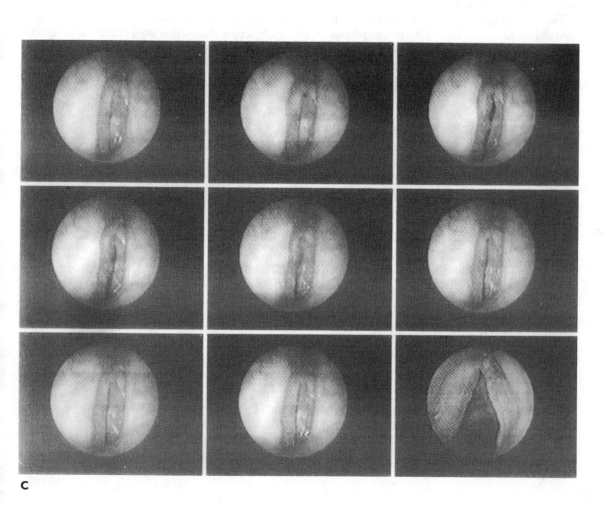

C

CARCINOMA OF THE VOCAL FOLD

Carcinomas are malignant neoplasms of unknown etiology. Cigarette smoking is closely related to the development of carcinoma of the larynx. Almost all carcinomas of the larynx are squamous cell carcinoma originating from the epithelium.

The lesion (Figure 6–13) is located in the epithelium and the superficial layer of the lamina propria in the very early stage, and, as it advances, it invades the vocal ligament and the muscle. The mechanical and aerodynamic correlates are similar to those in cases of papillomas. Vibratory behavior, therefore, is also similar to that discussed for cases of papillomas.

Carcinoma is much more frequently seen than papillomas. Very early carcinoma lesions sometimes cannot be differentiated from benign lesions under the traditional laryngeal mirror examination. A stroboscopic observation often enables us to detect a very small carcinoma because of the marked limitation of vibratory movements.

Carcinoma of the Vocal Fold (Unilateral)

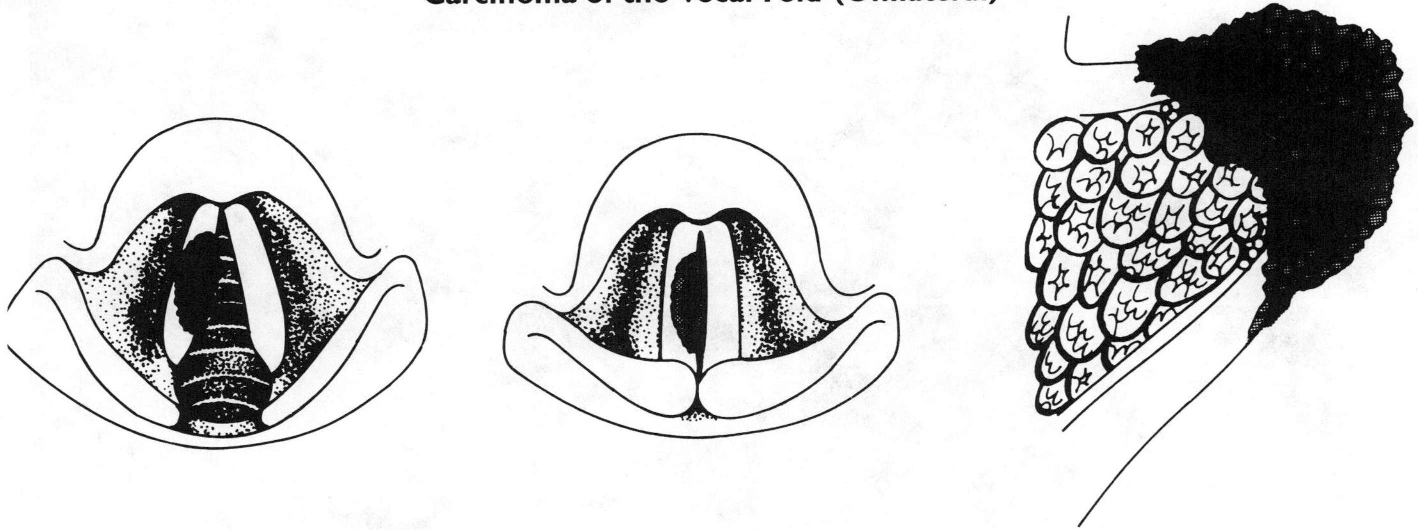

Location of pathology: *Epithelium* → *Lamina propria* → *Muscle* (*cover* → *body*)

Glottal incompetence: *Partly*

Symmetry: *Asymmetrical*

Homogeneity: *Heterogeneous*

Edge: *Nonlinear*

Length: Normal

Cover: Stiffness: *Increased* (markedly)

      Mass: *Increased*

Transition: Stiffness: *Often increased*

      Mass: *Often increased*

Body: Stiffness: *Occasionally increased*

      Mass: *Occasionally increased*

Obstacle: *Present*

Tonus of adductor muscles: Presumably often *increased*

Expiratory force: Presumably often *increased*

Subglottal pressure: Often *increased*

Figure 6–13. (A) Views of the larynx; a schematic of a frontal section of the vocal fold; and the mechanical and aerodynamic aspects of carcinoma of the vocal fold. (B) through (D) Videostroboscopic prints of a case of carcinoma of the vocal fold.

A

Figure 6-13 *(continued)*

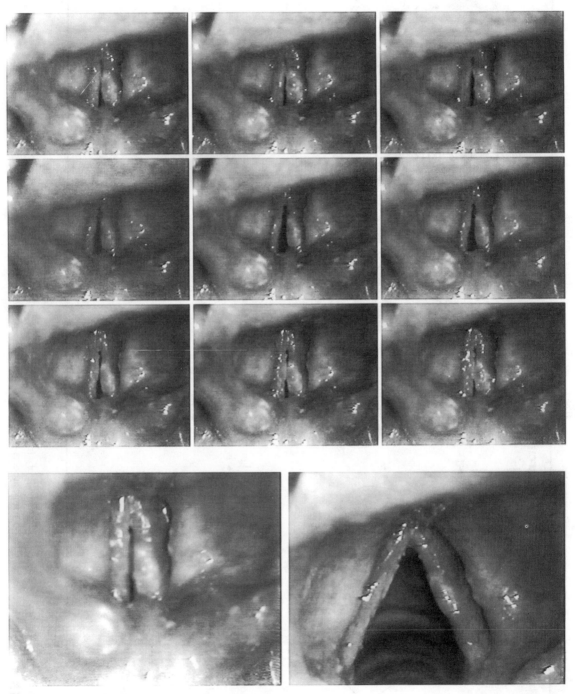

B

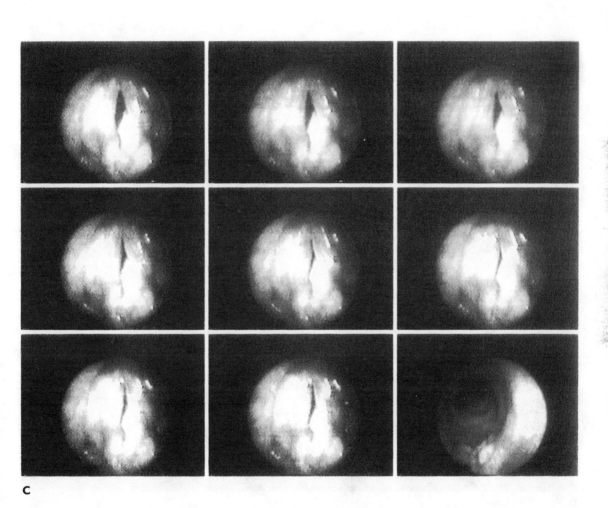

C

Figure 6–13 (continued)

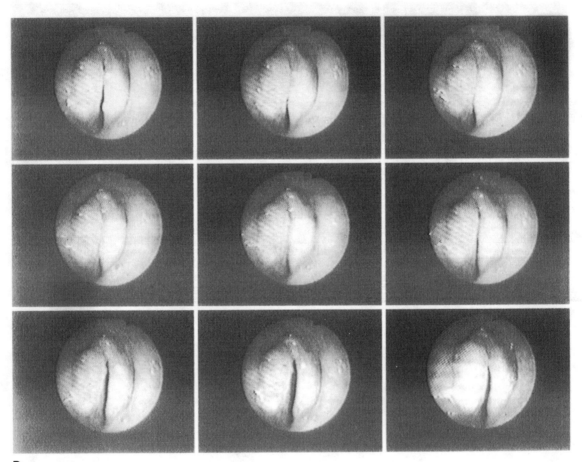

D

RECURRENT LARYNGEAL NERVE PARALYSIS

The recurrent laryngeal nerve innervates all intrinsic laryngeal muscles except for the cricothyroid muscle, which is innervated by the superior laryngeal nerve. Unilateral paralysis (Figure 6–14) is much more frequent than is bilateral paralysis.

The paralysis can be complete or incomplete. A complete paralysis is that in which all of the motor units in the recurrent laryngeal nerve are affected — as in the case of traumatic or surgical section of the nerve. The muscles are electrically silent or present only fibrillation potentials in EMG. An incomplete paralysis is that in which only some of the motor units in the nerve are affected — as in the case of neuritis or slight mechanical pressure on the nerve. The muscles present with voluntary electric potentials of a reduced number in EMG. In complete paralysis, the vocal fold not only is immobile but also has no muscular tonus. In incomplete paralysis, on the other hand, the vocal fold can be immobile or slightly mobile and it has some muscular tonus. Degrees of incomplete paralysis can vary.

Another classification of nerve paralysis is neuropraxia as opposed to axonotmesis and neurotmesis. The former is a temporary block of nerve impulse conduction and is reversible; a complete recovery can take place. The latter are associated with degeneration of the affected nerve fibers; regeneration of the nerve fibers can take place, but no complete recovery can be expected.

Whenever one treats a patient with recurrent laryngeal nerve paralysis, it is important to determine the degree and the nature of the paralysis. EMG is the best available clinical examination to obtain information about differential evaluation of these conditions. Stroboscopy, however, in the hands of a skilled examiner, can, with some limitations, be a substitute for EMG to obtain information about paralysis.

The pathology is located in the muscle. The glottis is usually not completely closed along its entire length; the glottal incompetence is often marked. The bilateral vocal folds are asymmetrical. The edge of the paralytic vocal fold is bowed when there is marked muscular atrophy. The stiffness and mass of the body are decreased to varying degrees, depending on the number of affected motor units. The tonus of the adductor muscles is also decreased to varying degrees.

The glottis usually does not close completely during vibrations. The movements of the bilateral vocal folds are asymmetrical and successive vibrations are aperiodic in some cases. The amplitude of horizontal excursion is frequently smaller on the paralytic side than on the unaffected side. The mucosal wave is often reduced or absent on the paralytic vocal fold. All these abnormalities in vibratory pattern tend to be more marked as the number of affected neurons increases. This is particularly true because the degree of disturbance of glottal closure and mucosal wave is frequently related to the number of the affected neurons, as evidenced by EMG findings (Fex & Elmqvist, 1973; Hirano, 1974; Schonharl, 1960a, b). Stroboscopy thus gives some valuable information for determining prognosis.

When the vocalis muscle is entirely atrophied and the vocal fold is thin and flaccid, the paralytic vocal fold presents with movements of a flag flapping in the wind. The unaffected vocal fold occasionally compensates by crossing the midline at the point of maximum closure when the edge of the paralytic vocal fold does not reach midline. More frequently, recruitment of the supraglottal structures to help increase medial compression can be seen by movement of the ventricular folds toward midline.

Recurrent Laryngeal Nerve Paralysis (Unilateral)

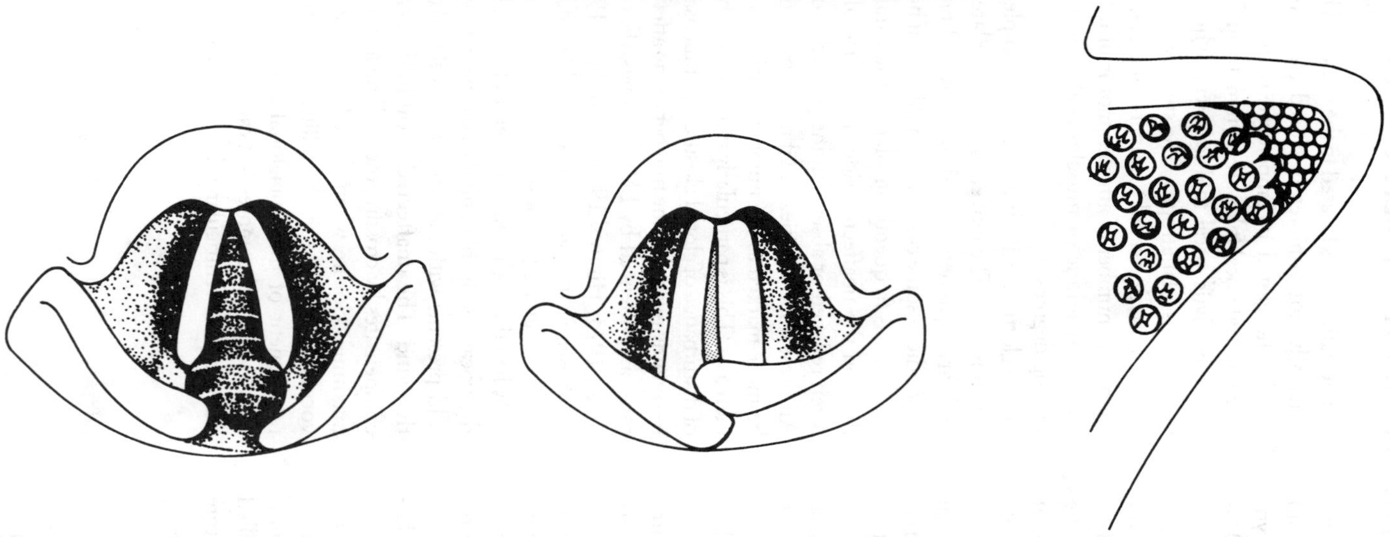

Location of pathology: *Muscle (body)*

Glottal incompetence: *Along entire length, marked*

Symmetry: *Asymmetrical*

Homogeneity: *Almost homogeneous*

Edge: *Bowed or linear*

Length: *Normal*

Cover: Stiffness: *Normal*

      Mass: *Normal*

Transition: Stiffness: *Normal*

           Mass: *Normal*

Body: Stiffness: *Decreased*

      Mass: *Decreased*

Obstacle: None

Tonus of adductor muscles: *Decreased, almost consistent*

Expiratory force: *Varying*

Subglottal pressure: *Varying*

A

Figure 6–14. (A) Views of the larynx; a schematic of a frontal section of the vocal fold; and the mechanical and aerodynamic aspects for unilateral com- plete nerve paralysis. (B) Videostroboscopic prints of a case of recurrent laryngeal nerve paralysis.

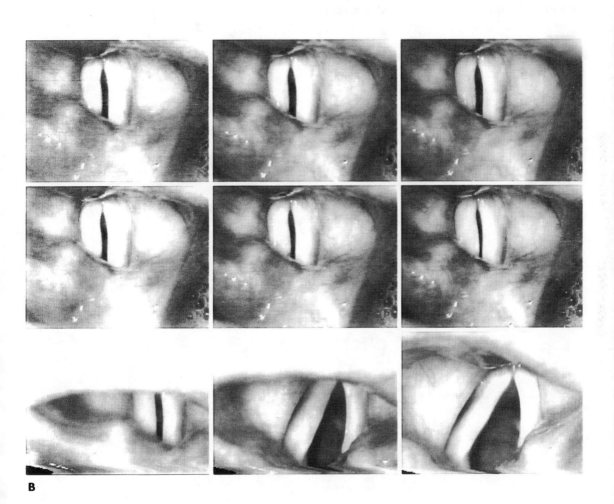

B

169

HYPERTROPHY OR MASS OF THE FALSE (OR VENTRICULAR) FOLD

When there is a marked hypertrophy or a large mass of the false vocal fold (ventricular fold), it interferes with vocal fold vibration. The lesion is usually unilateral (Figure 6–15).

The amplitude of horizontal excursion of the vocal fold on the affected side is decreased to varying degrees, and the vibratory movements are, therefore, asymmetrical between the two vocal folds. The mucosal wave on the affected side might be decreased.

Hypertrophy or Mass of the False Fold

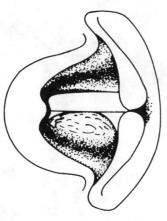

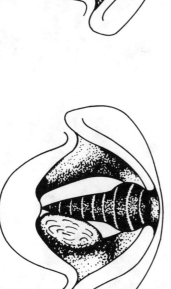

Location of pathology: *False Fold*

Glottal incompetence: None

Symmetry: *Symmetrical*

Homogeneity: Homogeneous

Edge: Linear

Length: Normal

Cover: Stiffness: Normal

Mass: Normal

Transition: Stiffness: Normal

Mass: Normal

Body: Stiffness: Normal

Mass: Normal

Obstacle: *Present*

Tonus of adductor muscles: Normal

Expiratory force: Normal

Subglottal pressure: Normal

Figure 6–15. (A) Views of the larynx; a schematic of the vocal fold; and the mechanical and aerodynamic aspects for hypertrophy or mass of the false fold. (B) through (E) Videostroboscopic prints of cases of hypertrophy and mass of the false fold.

A

Figure 6–15 *(continued)*

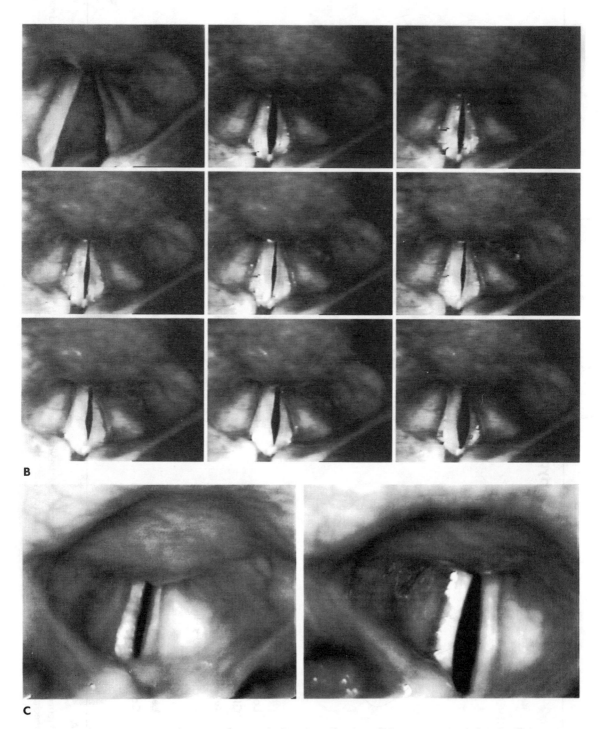

B

C

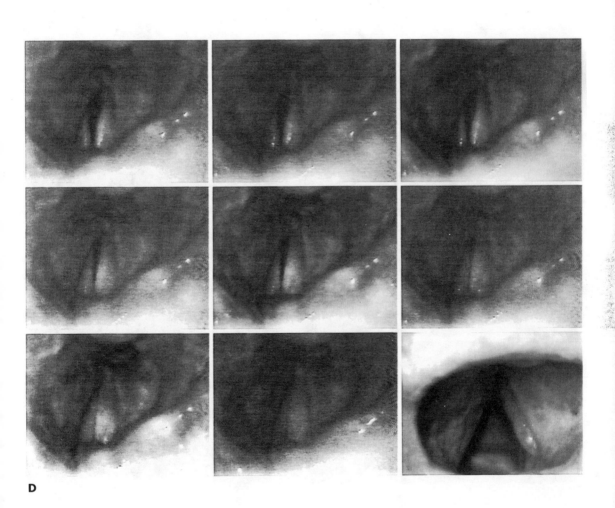

D

Figure 6–15 *(continued)*

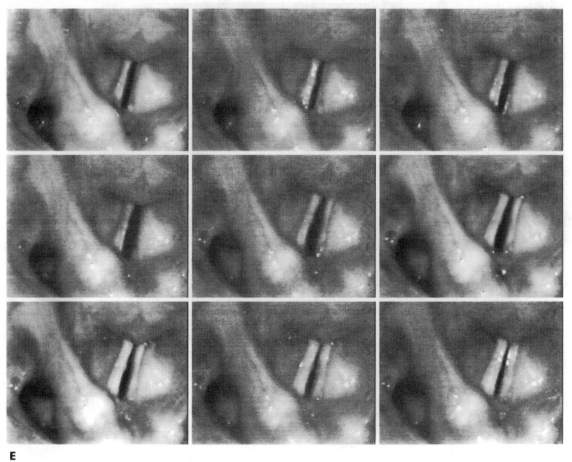

E

PROLAPSE OF THE VENTRICLE

The so-called "prolapse of the ventricle" consists of a swelling of the mucosa of the laryngeal ventricle. Occasionally, the mucosa of a lateral part of the upper surface of the vocal fold is also swollen. The lesion is usually unilateral. The etiology is unknown. When the lesion is small, there is no voice problem. If the lesion extends near the vocal fold edge, a slight degree of dysphonia is developed (Figure 6–16).

The vibratory movements of the vocal fold are somewhat limited on the affected side. The mucosal wave might be decreased. Vibratory movements of the two vocal folds are asymmetrical.

Prolapse of the Ventricle

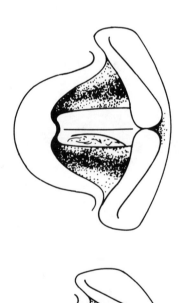

Location of pathology: *Upper surface of the vocal fold. Ventricle*
Glottal incompetence: None
Symmetry: Asymmetrical
Homogeneity: Almost homogeneous
Edge: Linear
Length: Normal
Cover: Stiffness: Normal
      Mass: Normal

Transition: Stiffness: Normal
      Mass: Normal
Body: Stiffness: Normal
      Mass: Normal
Obstacle: *Present*
Tonus of adductor muscles: Normal
Expiratory force: Normal
Subglottal pressure: Normal

A

Figure 6–16. (A) Views of the larynx; a schematic of the vocal fold; and the mechanical and aerodynamic aspects for so-called "prolapse of the ventricle." (B) and (C) Videostroboscopic prints of a case of prolapse of the ventricle.

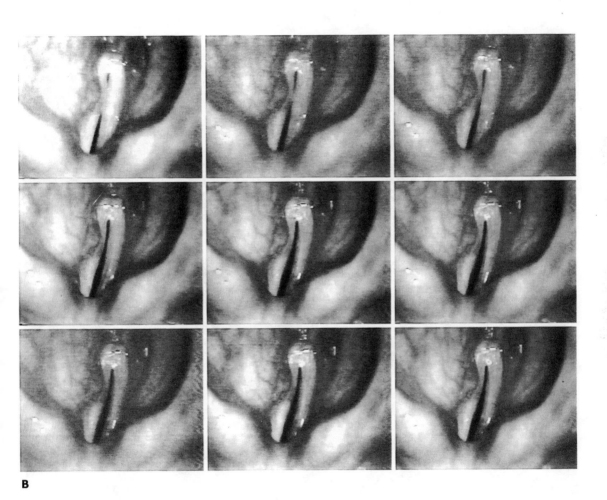

B

Figure 6–16 *(continued)*

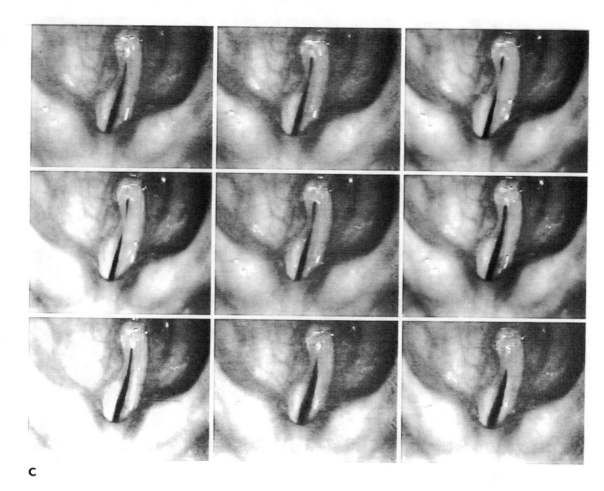

C

HYPERFUNCTIONAL (HYPERKINETIC) DYSPHONIA

Hyperfunctional dysphonia can be defined as a group of voice disorders that result from an excessive activity of the intrinsic and/or extrinsic laryngeal muscles during phonation (Figure 6–17). This condition can be associated with organic diseases, but there need not be any organic disease present. This description is limited to those hyperkinetic dysphonias that are purely functional in nature. In hyperfunctional dysphonia, the glottal closure is too tight. The false folds are often excessively adducted. The epiglottis is strongly pulled backward and the aryte-noids are markedly pulled forward during phonation. The vocal folds are often shortened. The mass of the whole layer structure of the vocal fold is increased. The stiffness of the cover and transition are variable, whereas that of the body is usually increased. The vocal fold covers and transitions are pressed against the opposing structure. The tonus of the adductor muscles is increased and so are the expiratory force and the subglottal pressure.

The closed phase of vibratory cycles is unusually long. The amplitude of horizontal excursion is small.

Hyperfunctional (Hyperkinetic) Dysphonia

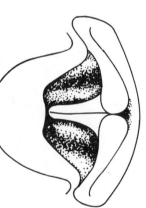
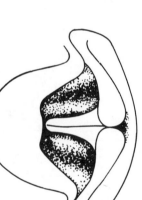
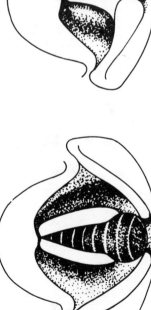
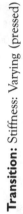

Location of pathology: No organic pathology

Glottal incompetence: None; *Too tight closure*

Symmetry: Symmetrical

Homogeneity: Homogeneous

Edge: Linear

Length: *Shortened*

Cover: Stiffness: *Varying (pressed)*

　　　　Mass: *Increased*

Transition: Stiffness: *Varying (pressed)*

　　　　　　Mass: *Increased*

　　Body: Stiffness: *Increased*

　　　　　Mass: *Increased*

　　Obstacle: None

Tonus of adductor muscles: *Increased*

Expiratory force: *Increased*

Subglottal pressure: *Increased*

A

Figure 6–17. (A) Views of the larynx; a schematic of the vocal fold; and the mechanical and aerodynamic aspects for hyperfunctional dysphonia. (B) through (D) Videostroboscopic prints of a case of hyperfunctional dysphonia.

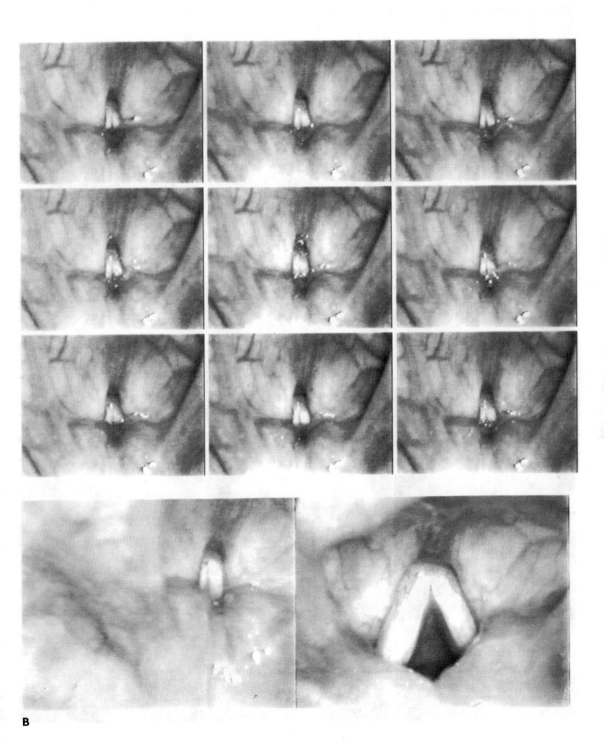

B

Figure 6–17 *(continued)*

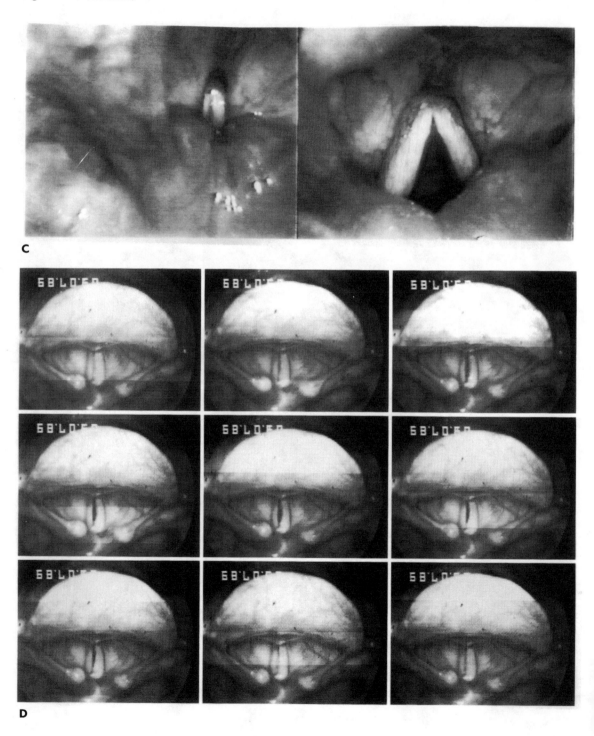

C

D

HYPOFUNCTIONAL (HYPOKINETIC) DYSPHONIA

Hypofunctional dysphonia refers to a group of voice disorders caused by an insufficient activity of the intrinsic and/or extrinsic laryngeal muscles during phonation (Figure 6–18). No organic disease is involved. The glottal closure is too weak, occasionally resulting in an incomplete closure. The stiffness of the body is decreased. The tonus of the adductory muscles, expiratory force, and subglottal pressure are also decreased.

The closed phase is short or nonexistent during vibratory cycles. The amplitude of horizontal excursion and the mucosal wave are decreased.

Hypofunctional (Hypokinetic) Dysphonia

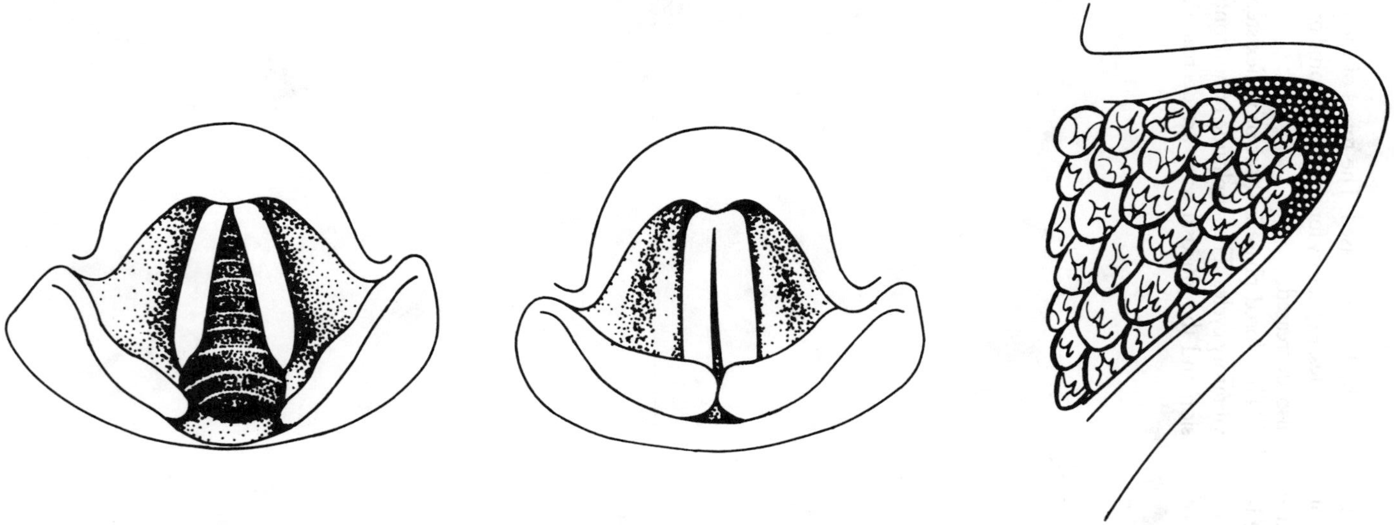

Location of pathology: No organic pathology

Glottal incompetence: Along entire length or none (loose closure)

Symmetry: Symmetrical

Homogeneity: Homogeneous

Edge: Linear

Length: Normal

Cover: Stiffness: Normal

Mass: Normal

Transition: Stiffness: Normal

Mass: Normal

Body: Stiffness: *Decreased*

Mass: Normal

Obstacle: None

Tonus of adductor muscles: *Decreased*

Expiratory force: *Decreased*

Subglottal pressure: *Decreased*

A

Figure 6–18. (A) Views of the larynx; a schematic of the vocal fold; and the mechanical and aerodynamic aspects for hypofunctional dysphonia. (B) and (C) Videostroboscopic prints of a case of hypofunctional dysphonia.

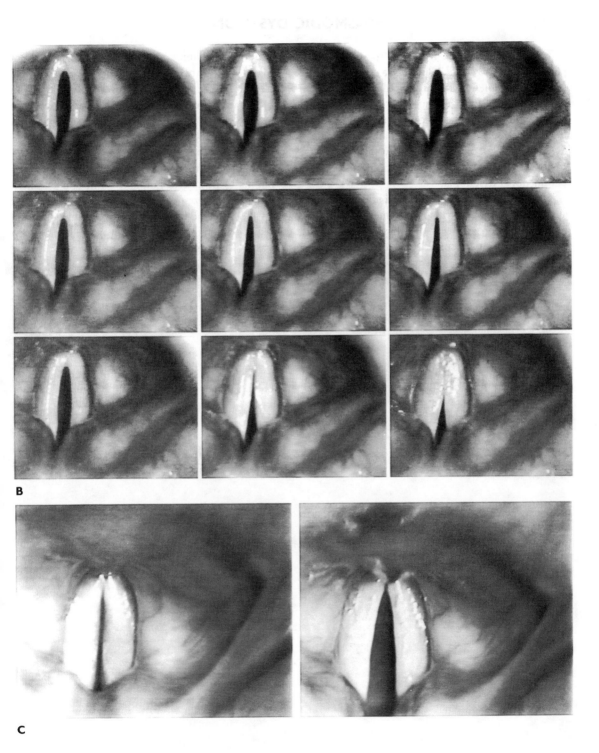

B

C

185

SPASMODIC DYSPHONIA

The etiology and the nature of spasmodic dysphonia are controversial. Clinically, a commonly observed phenomenon in this population is excessive glottal closure, with temporary releases repeated aperiodically during phonation (Figure 6–19). During the excessive closure, the mechanical and aerodynamic aspects of the phonatory mechanism is basically the same as that of an extreme case of hyperfunctional dysphonia.

The vibratory pattern of the vocal folds fluctuates aperiodically between that of extremely hyperfunctional phonation and that of a hypofunctional or normal phonation. In some instances, the vibratory characteristics might appear to be entirely normal, and in others vibration might appear normal except for an irregular twitching of the larynx or a continual tremor. In yet others, it might exhibit a combination of vibratory characteristics typically associated with other pathologies. This population is heterogeneous. Clinicians should not anticipate seeing one particular pattern; moreover, they should recognize that it is common even for people with severe spasmodic dysphonia to be able to normally produce a sustained tone. The aberrant vibratory characteristics might not be observable except during connected speech tasks or when the speaker has been stressed by such tasks as increased loudness.

Spasmodic Dysphonia

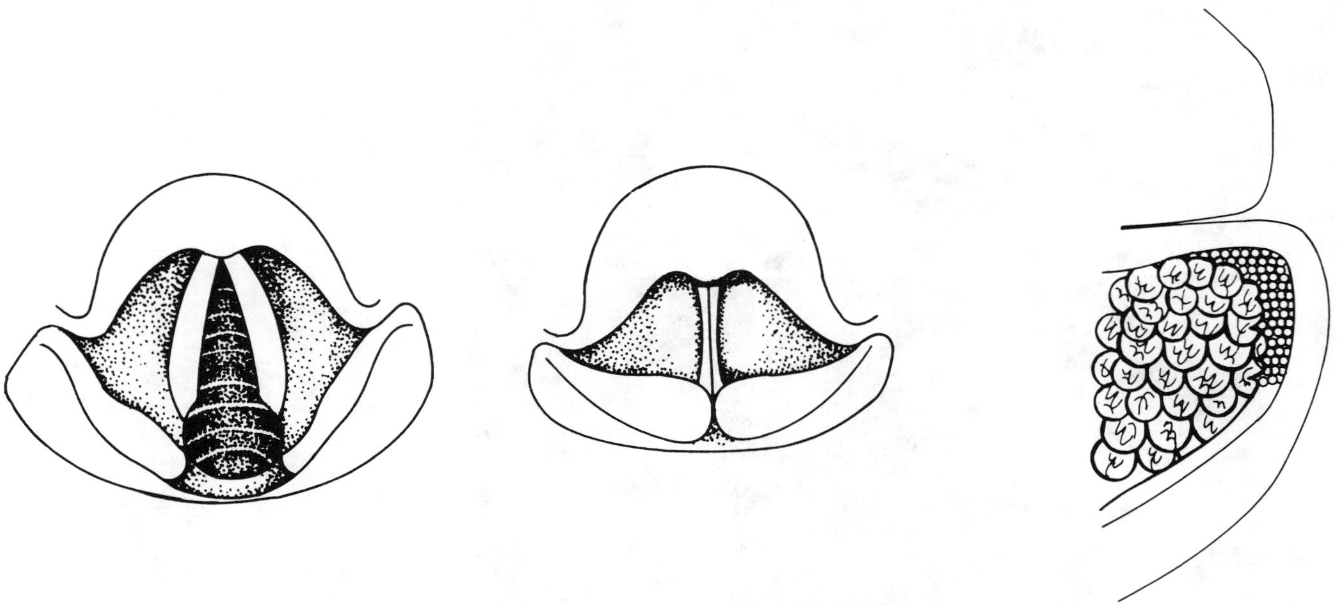

Location of pathology: No organic pathology

Glottal incompetence: None

Symmetry: Symmetrical

Homogeneity: Homogeneous

Edge: Linear

Length: Normal or shortened

Cover: Stiffness: Varying
Mass: Varying

Transition: Stiffness: Varying
Mass: Varying

Body: Stiffness: *Increased, fluctuating*
Mass: *Increased, fluctuating*

Obstacle: None

Tonus of adductor muscles: *Increased, fluctuating*

Expiratory force: *Increased, fluctuating*

Subglottal pressure: *Increased, fluctuating*

A

Figure 6–19. (A) Views of the larynx; a schematic of the vocal fold; and mechanical and aerodynamic aspects for spasmodic dysphonia. (B) Video-stroboscopic prints of a case of spasmodic dysphonia.

Figure 6–19 *(continued)*

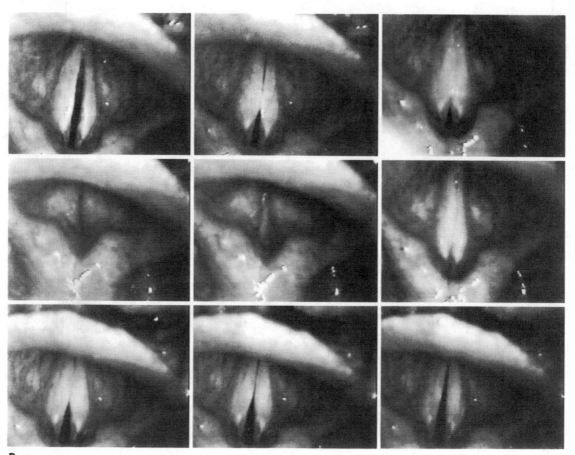

B

CONCLUSION

Understanding how stroboscopy can reveal various abnormalities and pathologies provides the clinician with a blueprint for making a diagnosis. Adding the results of other clinical data to stroboscopic data is the final step in using this visual perceptual tool.

STUDY QUESTIONS

1. Vibratory patterns of vocal pathologies depend on:

   a. Size, degree, and extent of lesion.

   b. Manner of phonation.

   c. Histological pattern of the disease.

   d. All of the above.

2. In catarrhal laryngitis, the mass of the cover is slightly increased resulting in:

   a. Greater fundamental frequency.

   b. Smaller fundamental frequency.

   c. Does not affect vocal fold vibration.

3. Abusive phonation can cause:

   a. A unilateral lesion.

   b. Subepithelial bleeding.

   c. A vocal fold nodule.

   d. Polypoid degeneration.

4. Reinke's edema:

   a. Usually occurs bilaterally.

   b. Results in decreased stiffness of the cover.

   c. Results in aperiodic vibrations of the vocal folds.

   d. All of the above.

5. The etiology of which of the following pathologies is unknown?

   a. Sulcus vocalis.

   b. Nodules.

   c. Epithelial hyperplasia.

   d. Papilloma.

6. Vocal fold scarring:

   a. Can be caused by trauma.

   b. Is always bilateral.

   c. Can be seen with the naked eye.

   d. None of the above.

7. Epithelial hyperplasia

   a. Originates from the epithelium and enters the superficial layer of the lamina propria.

   b. Is either congenital or acquired.

   c. Is common in women over 75.

   d. All of the above.

8. The only vocal fold lesion thought to be viral in origin is:

   a. Leukoplakia.

   b. Papilloma.

   c. Laryngeal web.

   d. Granuloma.

9. Recurrent laryngeal nerve paralysis affects all muscles of the larynx except the:

   a. Thyroarytenoid.

   b. Cricothyroid.

   c. Interarytenoid.

   d. None of the above.

10. Dysphonia can result from:

    a. Excessive activity of the intrinsic and extrinsic muscles of the larynx.

    b. Insufficient activity of the intrinsic and extrinsic muscles of the larynx.

    c. Swelling of the mucosa of the laryngeal ventricle.

    d. All of the above.

11. Vibratory characteristics of the vocal folds in patients with spasmodic dysphonia:

    a. Can be entirely normal.

    b. Can fluctuate between hyperkinetic and hypokinetic phonation.

    c. Can vary over time.

    d. All of the above.

CHAPTER

7

Relating Stroboscopy to Other Clinical Data

Voice is a complex phenomenon requiring multiple measures to describe its characteristics. Volumes have been written about its complexity. There currently is no clear consensus about what tests should be incorporated into daily clinical practice (National Institute for Deafness and other Communication Disorders Monograph, 1990). Nevertheless, clinics seem to agree that voice evaluation requires five basic steps: interviewing, observing, describing the voice, comparing observations to standards and normal values, and integrating information to determine treatment alternatives. It is sometimes necessary to use a variety of subjective and objective measures to complete these steps. Videostroboscopic recordings represent only one part — albeit an important part — of the laboratory examination. Relating videostroboscopy and the examination of vocal function to other laboratory examinations provides a full range of measures for voice evaluation.

INDICATIONS FOR LABORATORY TESTING

Instrumental techniques are used with increasing frequency to help describe the disordered voice. In-

dications for objective assessment of voice are controversial and center on three major issues: the necessity of testing, appropriateness of the tests, and the validity and reliability of the data. In fact, many otolaryngologists and speech pathologists hold fast to the belief that the ear and laryngeal mirror are the only tools needed, and that so-called "objective assessment" and the fancy instrumental "toys" that go with it are unnecessary. Others claim that the only instrument needed is the stroboscope because it is the only technique that provides a direct image of the larynx. Still others purport to be advocates of a multidimensional battery of tests that provide information on how the respiratory system interacts with the laryngeal system and that provide some measure of vocal quality, flexibility, endurance, physiological range, and effort.

Times change and needs are altered. The Voice Committee of the International Association of Logopedics and Phoniatrics — composed of otolaryngologists, speech pathologists, speech scientists, and phoniatrists — has recommended (1992) that it is no longer adequate to simply listen to the patient's voice and say, "The voice sounds better." To do so could be a disservice to a patient and to the person treating the dysphonia; it does not account for changes that might make phonation easier, as in improved glottal efficiency, does not provide an index of how much change has occurred or a prognostic indicator of how much additional change might be expected, does not address the need for augmentative treatment, and is subject to observer bias — particularly when judgments are being made by the clinician who provided the treatment.

Today, with the concept of accountability and the reality of litigation, it is necessary to objectively document the results of treatment and the potential for further change. Objective measures not only provide an unbiased documentation of change but also provide information that neither the eye nor the ear is capable of discerning. Thus, voice assessment is indicated pretreatment and posttreatment for all dysphonic patients, for patients whose diagnosis is questionable, and for those for whom decisions on the potential for change through behavioral management must be made. People with dysphonia secondary to acute laryngitis of short duration have nothing to gain from these objective measures.

Objective measures of vocal function include physical measures of the acoustic signal and physiological measures of the aerodynamic, movement, and electromyographic components of voice production. A test of vocal function is not appropriate if that test cannot answer questions about the presence of disease, the site or size of a lesion, the impact of the lesion on voice production, or the degree of vocal dysfunction — or if equally reliable information can be obtained by another, simpler procedure without discomfort or expense to the patient.

Because of the complexity of voice production, one generally cannot look at an isolated phenomenon without running the risk of misinterpreting the cause and effect of the dysphonia. Vocal function is like physical strength, which cannot be determined with any single scale or examination. Any vocal function test, however useful, can only partly evaluate vocal function. A battery of tests is needed for a full, valid, and reliable evaluation of the patient. This must include measurements of acoustic, aerodynamic, and movement parameters selectively applied and related to the auditory perceptual judgments of vocal quality, the visual perceptual judgments of vocal fold vibratory pattern, and appraisal of case history information that impacts voice production.

PRINCIPLES OF TEST SELECTION

Whatever vocal function tests are selected should be governed by the same basic principles that guide clinicians in the selection of stroboscopic instrumentation and procedures. Assessments should maximize the ability to measure voice during a variety of activities; provide repeated measures, reliable analysis, and unique data; and should be cost-effective. Every test should minimize restrictions on the vocal mechanism. Gottfried (1992) provides an excellent survey of the issues facing clinicians in test selection.

Sampling Adequacy

The test should provide an adequate sampling of the activity being investigated. A 1-sec sample of normal pitch and loudness provides no information about vocal performance at different pitch and loudness levels and no information during singing and, therefore, seems an inadequate sample to represent vocal function. Testing should include conditions that replicate typical habitual speaking and performance activities. Thus, when one is using the rigid endoscope, other additional testing that does not place restrictions on the speech mechanism becomes increasingly important.

Repeated Measures

If measurements are to be comparable from visit-to-visit and from institution-to-institution, it is crucial that both the same test protocol and the same recording procedures be used. Instructions, frequency, and other such conditions must be specified in patient records.

Measures of test performance should be based on precise, reliable methods and should be calibrated against reference standards. High precision in a laboratory procedure depends not only on careful attention to detail by the laboratory staff but also on maintaining consistent characteristics inherent in the methods and instrumentation. Tests must be done by qualified individuals (e.g., certified speech pathologists, speech scientists, or otolaryngologists) using properly calibrated and functioning equipment, and they must be done in precisely the same way every time.

Analysis

If tests are to be maximally useful, they must provide accurate, quantitative information. The same care one exercises in maintaining recording conditions from laboratory to laboratory must also be exercised in maintaining identical analyses. The decreasing cost of microcomputers should make this goal relatively easy to attain within even the most stringent budgets. Interpretations of analyzed data should be based on the most accurate models available that predict laryngeal function from relatively noninvasive movement, acoustic, and aerodynamic techniques.

When qualitative techniques such as videostroboscopy are used, it is important for both clinicians and patients to recognize that the resulting analyses are gross, are of unknown reliability, and are particularly subject to observer bias. Observers must be trained to look at the same details and to avoid observer bias caused by such factors as case history. This is also necessary in making objective measures. Care must be taken, too, to ensure that serial recordings are made under constant conditions.

Unique Information

A test should provide new information about the patient. It should not simply describe a condition in another way. Videostroboscopy can provide unique visual information not available from other measures. Aerodynamic studies provide information about respiratory support and the valving efficiency of the larynx; acoustic measures provide information about the physical properties of pitch, loudness, and variability; and EMG provides information about muscular integrity.

Cost Effectiveness

Economic factors cannot be disregarded when discussing tests and their interconnectedness, particularly when a new test is being considered for general use or when the laboratory must bear the cost of performing the procedure. Costs are based on the price of instruments and the complexity of the test; personnel time usually is the most important factor in determining cost. Tests are usually less expensive

when done by a designated person in the laboratory to enhance consistent simultaneous measurement. Ideally, tests that require minimum recording and analysis time would be emphasized. In the long run, however, the real cost of a procedure must be measured against the benefits it provides. Within reason, any test that might help preserve vocal longevity, prevent voice disorders, or enhance voice production should be considered worth the time, effort, and expense.

ROLE IN PHONOSURGERY

Tests of vocal function that help describe how the larynx operates have an important role in phonosurgical treatment. Whether made before or after surgery, these measures help address such questions as: Has the voice failed to improve because a surgery was inadequate or because the surgically corrected mechanism was being employed inappropriately? Do compensatory strategies adopted by the patient interfere with rehabilitation? Is the patient improved compared to self or to normal? How do age and sex influence the surgical outcome? What is the prognosis for decreased effort as a function of planned treatment?

Videostroboscopy can help answer these questions, but, used in isolation, it cannot provide vital information concerning cycle-to-cycle variation seen in perturbation analyses, information on intensity of production, or information on effort. What is needed is a laryngeal voice profile. Videostroboscopy does help explain why a person's voice breaks at high pitch or seems more effortful at low pitch.

Phonosurgery does not always result in a normal voice, and some gains might be too small to detect by listening or observing a videostroboscopic recording. Phonosurgery might change glottal efficiency but have no effect on voice production. The difference experienced by the patient might not be detected by listening or by observing the stroboscopic recordings, but might be noted in reduced airflow. Stroboscopic observations might not be possible on voices with severe irregularities of vibration. For those patients, valuable information would be gained from the acoustic measures of frequency, intensity, and time; from movement measures by EGG;

and by aerodynamic measures of airflow, air pressure, and air volume. Although these measures are indirect and require that clinicians must infer what is happening, information is provided on both the anatomical structure and the function of a larynx.

Successful treatment of a patient suffering from dysphonia depends on the clinician's ability to use a test battery to assess the type and degree of vocal impairment, to monitor the patient's subsequent progress throughout treatment, and to determine the type of treatment most likely to yield changes in voice quality, vocal efficiency, vocal effort, vocal loudness, or swallowing.

VOCAL FUNCTION TESTS

The noninvasive measurement techniques described in this chapter lead to a tangible record, can be done relatively quickly, and can be used as treatment probes to determine the role of different treatments, such as medialization procedures and voice therapy. In select cases — primarily paralysis and neurogenic disorders — invasive electromyographic and neurographic assessments are necessary.

Whether one is using videostroboscopy or other measures of vocal function, a primary object in describing the voice is to document habitual vocal behavior and vocal capabilities. In other words, the goal is to describe what the speaker does do and what the speaker can do with his or her laryngeal mechanism and to estimate what the speaker could do after either a surgical modification of the structure or voice therapy. This documentation of laryngeal function is used by clinicians for seven major purposes: (a) To help diagnose the voice problem; (b) to determine the cause or maintenance of the voice problem; (c) to document the degree and extent of causative disease and disturbance of phonatory function; (d) to help determine the best type of treatment; (e) to monitor treatment; and (f) to determine the prognosis.

The tests are conducted in a quiet environment under three conditions: (a) natural conversational speech; (b) phonatory tasks that test maximum performance and the flexibility of phonation; and (c) experimental treatment programs including manual compression of the thyroid alae. The experimental treatment tasks vary according to the patient's pathologic condition and phonatory pattern. Appendix 7-1 contains an example treatment probe list used for persons with glottic incompetence. These tests are done both with videostroboscopic light and during acoustic and aerodynamic measurements. The assumption is that if the techniques improve motion, airflow, frequency, intensity, or quality, they could be employed to change vocal function.

Generally, two baseline measurements for all tasks and measures are obtained to determine individual variability and to compare with posttreatment samples. The first baseline measurement is made during the initial evaluation, the second at a later time before treatment is begun. Clinicians model requested tasks to ensure that a patient understands what is being asked. Usually, three trials of each task are used to assess reliability of performance. Multiple trials are needed because patients with voice disorders frequently exhibit large trial-to-trial differences, which make posttreatment comparisons difficult unless pretreatment ranges are established. This variability can be seen in tasks produced at habitual levels as well as the extremes, and may be present across the test battery, including videostroboscopic measures. When practice effects are eliminated, large differences in performance from one token to the next provide important information about a patient's ability to control phonation.

The resultant measures from the test battery of multiple trials produced under different speaking conditions are used to determine seven major characteristics: (a) The frequency of the problem; (b) the duration of the problem; (c) the severity of the problem; (d) the effect of situation parameters (person, place); (e) the effect of specific phonetic contexts, pitches, and change in loudness; (f) variability as a function of the time of day and year; and (g) the interrelationship among measures such as the effect of compensatory strategies — seen from the strobe exam — on other measures of airflow, loudness, and contact time.

Clearly, laryngeal videostroboscopic examinations could not be practically applied to address these questions, underscoring again the need for multiparameter testing.

Normal Speaker Differences

Recognizing that differences exist in the normal population reduces the chance of misattributing normal variations in structure to functional deviations in the clinical population. Videostroboscopic observations are helpful in interpreting other measures. For example, a geriatric male with bowed vocal folds and low flows and air pressures would be interpreted to have poor respiratory support — a condition not uncommon with this age and gender. On the other hand, low flows from a 75-year-old male with a long closed phase and reduced mucosal wave could indicate a problem related more to hyperfunction than to poor respiratory support. A critical factor in making this interpretation would be knowledge of the norms in subglottal pressure and respiratory function measurements.

Normal variations related to age and gender are abundantly described in the literature. Studies of speakers with normal voice production and no complaints of voice problems or vocal fatigue have shown that normal speakers had vocal fold bowing, posterior glottal chinks, and a slight injection of the vocal folds. Functionally, the greatest differences were seen between males and females, children and adult males, and young adults and geriatrics. These changes are consistent with biological changes occurring elsewhere in the body (Figure 7–1). Stroboscopic observations showed males generally had longer closed phase and more complete glottic closure than females did, children had a larger posterior chink and shorter closed phase than adult males did, and geriatrics had more asymmetry and lower amplitude of vibration than their younger counterparts did. Aerodynamic studies show slightly higher flows in males, and intra-oral pressures changing as a function of age, with the greatest pressures exhibited by young children and the lowest by geriatrics. Intensity measures show similar trends. These findings are interpreted to mean that children have greater respiratory support and closing force. Failure to consider these normal variations related to life span changes can lead to erroneous clinical judgments about laryngeal structure and function (Figure 7–2).

It would be foolhardy to assume that the wide range of differences among normal speakers does not occur with the same or even greater frequency among speakers with various pathologic conditions of the larynx. Because of the wide range of anatomical and physiological differences among speakers and because of speakers' differing abilities to compensate for deficits, there is no strict one-to-one correspondence between observed changes in the vibratory pattern and existing pathologic conditions, or in the observed pattern's relation to other measures. Nevertheless, there are strong trends. Measures usually fit together like a puzzle, with one piece leading to the natural connection of the next and together providing a picture that cannot be visualized with data from only one of the parts.

Acoustic Analysis

The acoustic output of the vocal mechanism provides a physical link between the events associated with the production and perception of sound (Weismer, 1984). Acoustic voice analysis has a long history and is one of the best understood forms of voice analysis. Acoustic signal analysis provides an indirect measure of the vibratory patterns of the vocal folds, as well as vocal tract shapes and changes in those shapes over time (Laver, Hillers, & Mackenzie, 1992). Measurements include various derivatives of frequency, intensity, and time. Interpretation of the data is made relative to normative data bases and is subject to changes based on age, sex, type of phonation, and voice training. The analysis is done during sustained phonation tasks and during continuous speech.

Voice treatment is indicated for individuals with reduced vocal range, low signal-to-noise ratio (SNR), fundamental frequency incompatible with age or sex, inappropriate habitual intensity level, high perturbation scores, inappropriate vocal tract configuration, and inconsistency between habitual performance and potential performance. Combining acoustic measures and videostroboscopic measures is an ideal marriage; the stroboscopic images help explain the source of the acoustic findings; the acoustic results help quantify the movements qualitatively observed with the stroboscope.

Frequency

Frequency is the physical correlative of the perceptual phenomenon of pitch. It represents the num-

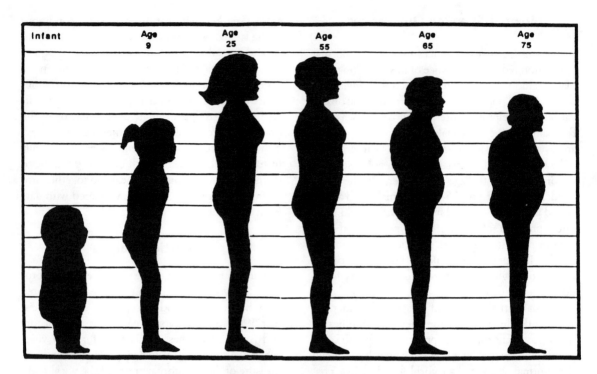

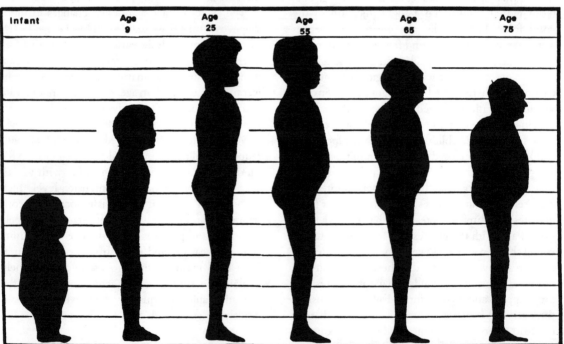

Figure 7–1. Variations in normal voice production are consistent with other biological characteristics.

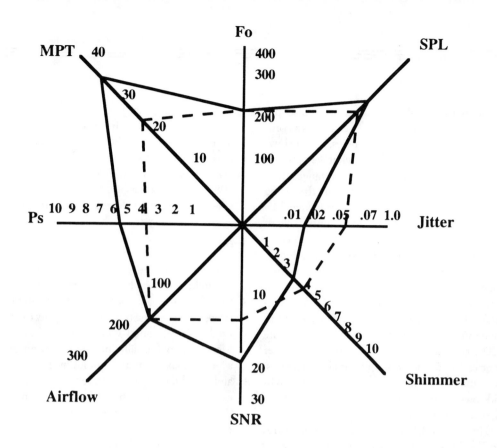

A

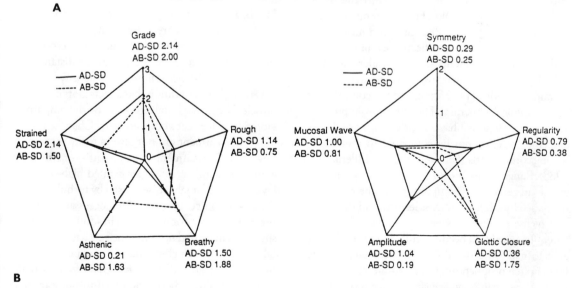

B

Figure 7–2. (A) Polar graphs of measures of vocal function show children are louder and use greater respiratory support. Subglottal pressure is higher and maximum phonation time longer. (B) Polar graphs display selected stroboscopic observations of perceptual measures for two groups with spastic dysphonia.

ber of times the vocal folds open and close per second and is measured in hertz. The voice is a complex tone comprising many frequencies, but the lowest fundamental frequency (F_o) is what we perceive as the vocal pitch. In normal speakers it ranges from less than 60 Hz for the basso voice to more than 1568 Hz for the soprano voice. Frequency is changed by altering laryngeal tension and is done continually to provide the changes necessary for singing and communication. Most speakers are able to produce a wide range of frequencies above and below their fundamental frequency. As the pitch is elevated, stroboscopic images show that the vocal folds elongate, the cover becomes stiffer, and both the amplitude and mucosal wave become reduced (see Figure 7–2). The converse pattern is present at the lower frequencies where the closed phase also increases.

Phonation range is the range spanned by the highest and lowest frequencies a patient can produce. Young adults have a frequency range of 2½ to 3 octaves (Bless, 1988; Colton, 1972; Hirano, 1981a; Orlikoff & Baken, 1990), which is 30 to 36 semitones, and geriatrics have a frequency range of 2 octaves or less. The ability to produce a large frequency range demands neuromotor control, adequate respiratory support, and the ability to modify the shape and length of the vocal folds. Frequency range is easy to measure in the clinic. Because it is a measure of extremes, frequency range reflects the limits of laryngeal adjustments. Patients show considerable individual differences, which are related to factors such as training, mode of phonation, and the condition of the anatomical structure. The variation is predictable. Singers typically have a wide range at all ages and, therefore, cannot be compared to their nonsinging counterparts (Peppard, Bless, & Milenkovic, 1988). Range increases until early adulthood and decreases in geriatrics. The upper end of the register is decreased by edema and mass lesions, and the lower end of the register is extended by Reinke's edema when the vocal fold becomes fuller and is no longer able to make the shape changes necessary for the higher pitch productions, Repeated measures of frequency range can provide a simple means of following the treatment of selected disorders.

The long-term variability of fundamental frequency, or pitch sigma, refers to the standard deviation of fundamental frequency during speech. It is not to be confused with jitter, which is a short-term measure of the variability of cycle-to-cycle variation in voice. The pitch sigma of both adult males and females ranges between 2 and 4 semitones (Baken, 1987; Colton & Casper, 1990; Hirano, 1981a; Linville & Fisher, 1985; Mysak, 1959; Stoicheff, 1981).

Intensity

Intensity relates to loudness as frequency relates to pitch; it is the physical correlate of the perceptual phenomenon, and it reflects the amplitude or strength of the tone produced. Intensity can be measured from sustained vowels or connected speech. Measurements usually include the mean or overall average, maximum and minimum levels, and variability. Obtaining accurate, repeatable measures necessitates the replication of mouth-to-microphone distance, speech task, frequency, and noise characteristics. There are several commercially available, easy-to-use sound-level meters or analyzers, and computer programs than run on IBM®-compatible and Macintosh® systems. Normal individuals should have an intensity range of no less than 30 dB, a maximum level of about 110 dB, a habitual level of 70 to 75 dB, and an intensity sigma of 4 to 6 dB. Sound level measurements are dependent on the distance between the speaker's mouth and the microphone. Intensity is reduced by the square of distance, so doubling the distance will reduce intensity by 3 dB. Any pathologic condition that affects glottal closure, muscle force, subglottal pressure, or the amplitude vibration will affect vocal intensity. Changes resulting from treatment are not always easily measured, however. Pretreatment, open glottis or irregular glottis frequently creates exaggerated high-intensity levels that are largely noise caused by turbulent air at the glottal source. It is, therefore, necessary to measure overall quality or noise level in addition to intensity. With increased noise, as one gets with poor glottal closure, a rough glottal margin, and perturbation, the signal is degraded. Even though the voice sounds loud the quality is poor, the signal-to-noise ratio is low, and speech intelligibility may be impaired.

Videostroboscopic recordings show increased amplitude of movement, and increased vertical dimensions in the mucosal wave with increases in intensity. The closed phase also increases.

Physiological Frequency Range of Phonation

The physiological frequency range of phonation (PFRP) is determined by having the speaker produce his or her frequency range at maximum and minimum intensity levels. The range is expressed in semitones. The resultant frequencies are plotted against intensities to yield a PFRP. PFRP is said to reflect the physiological limits of a person's voice. Professional voice users generally have considerably larger PFRP territories than typical speakers and typical speakers cover greater ranges than do speakers with voice disorders. As a clinical measure, the frequency/intensity profile can provide the most consistent evidence of change resulting from treatment.

Perturbation

Acoustic perturbations describe the random deviations from complete regularity of cycle-to-cycle movements. These movements can be quantified with any number of software programs and have thus become fashionable as voice laboratories report. Cycle-to-cycle movements are never completely regular (Baken, 1987; Boves, 1984; Laver, Hiller, & Mackenzie, 1988). The random variability of the cycle-to-cycle duration is called jitter and amplitude is termed shimmer. Jitter and shimmer are thought to contribute to the rough perceptual quality called harshness. When great enough they also contribute to irregular appearance in vibration in the stroboscopic image. The etiology of the abnormal movement patterns can be from hyperkinetic muscle adjustments, from the mechanical consequences of neoplastic growth, or from impairments to the neural integrity of the system. Generally speaking, the greater the magnitude of the lesion, glottal gaps, irregular margin, or neural impairment, the greater the perturbation factor. In some voice problems the perturbation is constant; in others it occurs at the onset or termination of phonation or when lung volume is not sufficiently high to overdrive and compensate for the underlying laryngeal deficits. Perturbations are also related to changes in age, frequency, and intensity. In general, the greater the tension is on the vocal folds, the lower the perturbation is. Thus, geriatric speakers with flaccid folds speaking at a low F_o would have more perturbation than a young adult speaking with a loud voice. The low level of perturbation present in all speakers is not seen under stroboscopic observation. The higher levels associated with pathology contribute to a distorted image.

Aerodynamic Measures

Aerodynamics refers to the average air pressures, air flows, and air volume produced as part of the peripheral mechanics of the respiratory, laryngeal, and supralaryngeal airways.

As such, clinical measures of airflow, air pressure, and air volume are thought to reflect laryngeal valving efficiency and respiratory support. These indirect measures of vocal function change as a function of the opening and closing patterns of the vocal folds and as a function of respiratory support and should be used to supplement acoustic, glottal kinematic, and other measures of vocal function.

Quantitative aerodynamic measures tend to follow a dichotomy between gross and fine characteristics (as do acoustic measures; e.g., Scherer, Gould, Titze, Meyers, & Sataloff, 1988). Measures of gross characteristics are taken over a few hundred milliseconds or more. Examples are average subglottal pressure, average airflow, calculated flow resistance (subglottal pressure divided by airflow), subglottal aerodynamic power (subglottal pressure times flow), acoustic efficiency (output power divided by subglottal aerodynamic power), sound pressure level, and other measures or derived variables dealing with average or integrated values. On the other hand, fine measures of aerodynamic characteristics deal with short-term calculation on the order of tens of milliseconds or less and often deal with such aspects of pressures and flows within individual phonatory cycles. These measures deal with characteristics of the glottal flow as peak values, slopes at specific times, relative delays, dynamic (time varying) subglottal pressure and vocal tract pressures, and intraglottal pressures. Aerodynamic characteristic measures also are associated with specific vibratory motions of the vocal folds as well as spectral details, though the precise association is still not well understood.

During the sustained production of vowels, high airflows indicate poor laryngeal valving, and low airflows suggest hyperfunction, obstruction, low effort, or poor respiratory support. Low airflows coupled with a loud voice and normal or high intraoral pressures help rule out poor respiratory support and reduced effort. Similarly, high glottal resistance indicates excessive closure resulting from an obstruction. Musculoskeletal tension, stiff structure, associated compensatory movements, and low glottal resistance indicate an incomplete approximation of the vocal folds. Airflows and air pressures are particularly useful in resolving issues concerned with closure on different planes. For example, glottal closure might appear complete from stroboscopic recordings but accompanying low resistance and high airflow — incompatible with such closure findings — would lead clinicians to further testing, such as radiographic studies of the structure.

Airflow Rate

Airflow rate refers to the volume velocity of air moving through the glottis, and in normal subjects can cover a large range. A critical range would appear to be approximately 40 to 200 cm^3 (Hirano, 1981a) (see also Kitajima, 1985; Wilson & Star, 1985, who suggest wider ranges), and when used alone, is not often a clinically sensitive measure. The mean flow rate appears to be relatively high in many cases of recurrent laryngeal nerve paralysis and large tumors (Hirano, 1981a) and low in cases of hyperfunction. Mean flow rate can be useful in following treatment of the larynx if significant changes are made in glottal competency. The primary worth of the mean flow rate, however, is probably in conjunction with subglottal pressure in measures of glottal resistance and subglottal aerodynamic power.

The inverse filtered flow at this time is clinically useful and should be incorporated as a routine procedure as its technology and accuracy continue to be studied. Measures of peak flow, peak derivative flow, bias offset flow, speed quotient, and open quotient are highly relevant to voice quality, vibratory motion of the vocal folds, and glottal adduction.

Glottal Resistance

When airflow values are divided into subglottal pressure, the measure is glottal resistance. Glottal resistance is more informative regarding glottal competence than is either flow or pressure means used alone. This is interpreted to mean that more clinicians should be using glottal resistance measures. High resistances are present in hyperfunction, spasmodic dysphonia, and some obstructive pathologies, and relates to a long closed phase in videostroboscopic recordings.

Subglottal Pressure

The technique of interest at the moment for both clinical and research purposes is the estimation of subglottal pressure from measurements of oral pressure (Lofqvist, Carlborg, & Kitzing, 1982; Rothenberg, 1973; Smitheran & Hixon, 1971; Shipp, 1973) In this procedure, a CVC string such as /pip/, /pæp/, or /bæp/ is repeatedly produced during a single exhalation by the subject or patient in a legatto (smooth) manner. When the lips close for the bilabial consonant, the glottis opens to produce the voiceless consonant. The pressure below the vocal folds during the vowel production is communicated to the oral cavity as the air flows from the trachea. The estimate of subglottal pressure is taken from a measure of the oral pressure during the consonant closure. This particular technique is indirect but relatively accurate. (Lofqvist, Carlborg, and Kitzing [1982] found an average difference from direct measures of subglottal pressure of 0.85 mm H$_2$O.) It is also relatively simple, and, if airflow is also measured during the vowel portion, an estimate of glottal resistance can be obtained. The task can be used with patients who can completely occlude the oral airway so that airflow from the trachea quickly creates pressure equilibration. If the syllable rate is too slow, there is the risk of respiratory pumping during the consonant closures, giving oral pressures greater than the subglottal pressures during the vowel. If the syllable rate is too fast, there may be not enough time for the oral pressure to build up to the value of the subglottal pressure. Smitheran and Hixon (1971) propose a rate of 1.5 syllables per second.

The relationships between these aerodynamic measures of average airflows and average air pressures and clinical needs are not straightforward. Like stroboscopy, changes of pressures and flows can be examined over time for a patient undergoing phonatory change or for posttreatment checks. For example, phonosurgery often changes the adductory nature of the larynx, and relatively large changes in airflows and air pressures and derived measures of glottal resistances and subglottal power may occur. Also, for example, regaining steadiness of the voice as a result of botulinum toxin (Botox) treatment in patients with spasmodic dysphonia can be monitored by using the patient's average airflow during sustained vowels.

From a clinical point of view, subglottal pressure threshold measurement (Titze, 1988) that allows the vocal folds to just begin oscillation is important. Lower threshold pressures would correspond to less expiratory work to phonate, thus allowing phonation (and speaking) to feel easier.

The fundamental frequency of the voice depends primarily on the tension per cross-sectional area of the vocal fold tissue and the vocal fold length (Titze, 1988). In addition, the subglottal pressure plays a significant role in the change of fundamental frequency especially for lower frequencies. As the subglottal pressure increases, the lateral extension of the vocal folds in each of the vibratory cycles is increased, which increases the effective length and tension of the vocal folds (Titze, 1989). This raises the pitch. This frequency control through subglottal pressure change may contribute strongly to intonation control during speaking.

Many studies have indicated that intensity increases as subglottal pressure increases (e.g., Isshiki & Ringel, 1964; Iwata, 1988; Ladefoged & McKinney, 1963). Titze and Sundberg (1992) show that glottal geometry (glottal adduction, vocal fold medial convergence, vocal fold medial shape, and the vertical phasing of the vocal folds) also may play a significant role in intensity control. The cyclic airflow just above the glottis is the signal affected by the subglottal pressure and intracycle glottal movements, and is the signal by which acoustic intensity is obtained.

If changes due to treatment of the voice are relatively subtle but meaningful, as is the case for many nonsurgical voice problems of quality, comfort, ease, and endurance, average values of aerodynamic aspects of the voice may be insufficient to reflect those changes. There is a large variability for airflow across patients as well as within a particular patient (Bless & Hirano, 1982), and clinically relevant changes may be buried in this variability. Also, important measures like glottal flow resistance may not correspond well to clinical voice quality judgments (Holmberg & Leanderson, 1983). The detection of phonatory changes and accurate mapping to diagnostic categories and voice qualities may require finer analysis. Measures of subtle voice change, smaller measurement error, and a strong connection to phonatory theory are required (Scharer, 1984).

The fine level of aerodynamic assessment consists of specific, instantaneous, cyclic measures of subglottal and supraglottal pressure and the glottal volume velocity signal obtained through inverse filtering of the output of oral air airflow. This technique yields measures that can provide meaningful characterization of subtle changes in voice related to vibration and vocal fold morphology.

Electromyographic (EMG) Assessment

EMG is useful for making diagnostic and prognostic decisions about neuromuscular diseases and functional disorders. It is used to study the action of muscles in vivo (kinesiology) and to diagnose neuromuscular pathologies. It is the only procedure that directly samples muscular activity.

The presence or absence of six features of EMG — electrical silence, fibrillation potentials, polyphasic potentials, high-amplitude potentials, normal potentials but reduced number, and normal potentials — helps clinicians make diagnostic decisions. EMG can help to differentiate laryngeal nerve paralysis from central neurologic disorders, from functional disorders, and from arytenoid fixation. EMG results also may have prognostic value in cases of vocal fold paralysis. Stroboscopic studies can demonstrate that these structures are not moving normally, but they cannot discern the etiological bases.

INTEGRATING LABORATORY MEASURES

Symptoms and treatment objectives both depend on the shape, tension, size, surface, and the speaker's control of the vocal folds, all of which can be described from a combination of instrumental measures. Quantitative and qualitative measures are compared to age- and sex-based norms. It is impossible to mention here all the potential dysphonic combinations of normal and abnormal values that are clinically useful. Normal physiological changes with age include reductions in mean airflow, air pressure, phonation time, signal-to-noise ratio, maximum performance tasks, vital capacity and other lung partition measures, changes in the morphological appearance of the larynx, changes in vocal quality, and an increase in the dryness of the mucosa, which results in poorer vibratory source. In general, clinicians look for results that point to incomplete glottal closure, excessive glottal closure, problems of motor control, problems of stiff or immobile structures, problems with changes in tissue characteristics or mechanical properties of the vocal folds, or inconsistency in the physiological use of the mechanism. If these signs are inconsistent as aids to making decisions about appropriate treatment, clinicians use the patient's history and other examination results to exclude psy-

chological, neurological, or other medical problems that might contribute to the dysphonia. After treatment, the battery of tests is repeated to measure the change and monitor the success. Assessments also might be helpful in identifying those treatment techniques that work best and in aiding clinical scientists in developing better treatments.

Voice is reevaluated at the conclusion of each treatment protocol to determine if improvement has been satisfactory. Minimal tests should include baseline comparisons of aerodynamic acoustic with auditory and visual-perceptual judgments of voice production. If voice problems persist, additional tests might be needed. If improvement is satisfactory, the patient can be dismissed from treatment and be seen in follow-up examinations. If improvement is unsatisfactory, the clinician uses laboratory tests in an attempt to determine the reason for dissatisfaction and either initiates new therapy or refers the patient to other health care professionals for additional tests or treatment.

Thus, we see that laboratory assessment of voice is the study of biomechanical, neuromuscular, and aerodynamic processes involved in sound production. No single measure is adequate to characterize the problems presented. Stroboscopic examination provides one critical part of the puzzle of vocal function.

Treatment Probe List for Glottic Incompetence

	Increase orality	Relaxation	Change of vowel	Change of onset	Muscle strengthening	Pitch change	Loudness change	Digital manipulation	Change of breathing	Change of posture
ELIMINATION OF DISORDER										
BEHAVIORAL										
Normal voice										
Improved quality										
Pitch improved										
Loudness improved										
Tension reduced										
PERCEPTUAL										
Auditory: Voice improved on any parameter										
Visual: Vibration improved on any parameter										
Effort level reduced										
Patient accepts voice										
AERODYNAMIC										
Decreased airflow										
Increased airflow										
Change in R_G										
Increase in V										
Increase in control										

(continued)

	Increase orality	Relaxation	Change of vowel	Change of onset	Muscle strengthening	Pitch change	Loudness change	Digital manipulation	Change of breathing	Change of posture
ACOUSTIC										
Frequency range increased										
Habitual frequency age-sex appropriate										
Intensity range increased										
Habitual intensity situation appropriate										
Jitter decreased										
Shimmer decreased										
SNR increased										
VOICE EDUCATION										
Know how to best use voice										
Know voice limitations										
Know how to avoid voice problems										

STUDY QUESTIONS

1. Which of the following is not part of a typical voice evaluation:

   a. Interview.

   b. Demanding the patient change his/her vocal habits.

   c. Describing and observing vocal behaviors/ parameters.

   d. Comparing observations to standards and normative values.

2. Instrumental techniques are used to promote an objective assessment including:

   a. Providing an unbiased documentation of change.

   b. Providing information that neither the eye nor the ear is capable of discerning.

   c. Removing the accountability of the speech pathologist.

   d. a and b.

3. A reliable vocal function evaluation consists of: (Choose all that apply.)

   a. One vocal function test of the clinician's choice.

   b. Stroboscopy.

   c. A battery of tests including acoustic, aerodynamic, and stroboscopic evaluation.

   d. Auditory and visual perceptual judgments.

4. Vocal function test selection should take into consideration whether the test:

   a. Measures voice during a variety of tasks.

   b. Provides repeated measures.

   c. Is cost effective.

   d. Provides reliable and unique data.

5. Stroboscopy also can aid in phonosurgical therapy by:

   a. Comparing pre- and post-treatment vocal fold conditions.

   b. Noting any compensatory strategies the patient has adopted.

   c. Giving information on cycle-to-cycle variation.

   d. a and b.

6. Vocal function measures are conducted under which of the following conditions:

   a. Natural conversational speech.

   b. Phonatory tasks testing maximum performance.

   c. Experimental treatment protocols.

   d. All of the above.

7. Multiple trials of the vocal function measures are used to determine which of the following: (Choose all that apply.)

   a. Frequency of the problem.

   b. Duration of the problem.

   c. Severity of the problem.

   d. Effect of situation.

   e. Patient personality.

8. Normally, there are differences between speakers on vocal parameters, but there are some consistent differences between males and females, males and children, and young adults and geriatrics. Which of the following statements are *true*?

   a. Women have longer closed phases than men.

   b. Children have a larger posterior glottal chink than adult males.

   c. Geriatrics have more symmetry than their younger counterparts.

   d. None of the above.

9. Acoustic analysis provides a measure of frequency, intensity, and time of the vibratory patterns of the vocal folds. Which of the following must be taken into consideration in the interpretation of the data?

a. Age.

b. Gender.

c. The phonatory task.

d. Voice training.

e. Time of day.

10. Frequency, the physical correlative of pitch, is changed by altering laryngeal tension. As pitch is elevated, which of the following is *not* true?

a. Vocal folds elongate.

b. The cover becomes more stiff.

c. Amplitude increases.

d. Mucosal wave is reduced.

11. Reductions in the upper end of the phonation range often occur with:

a. Edema.

b. Nodules.

c. Polyps.

d. All of the above.

12. Perturbation measures are *not* affected by changes in:

a. Gender.

b. Age.

c. Frequency.

d. Intensity.

13. During sustained production of vowels, high airflow measures can indicate:

a. Poor laryngeal valving.

b. Possible laryngeal pathology.

c. Poor respiratory support.

d. a and b.

14. Electromyography is useful for making diagnostic and prognostic decisions about:

a. Neuromuscular disease.

b. Laryngeal nerve paralysis versus central neural disorders.

c. Vocal fold paralysis.

d. All of the above.

APPENDIX

Instructions for Making a Zoetrope

INSTRUCTIONS FOR MAKING ZOETROPE

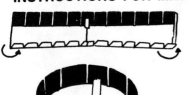

CUT ALONG THIS EDGE

1. Carefully cut pages from this book.

2. Paste the circle onto a piece of thick cardboard or foamcore and cut out.

3. Cut out the two strips labeled zoetrope sides. Tape the strips together at B being careful not to occlude a slit. Fold up the bottom tabs.

4. Tape the ends of the strip together to form a ring with the tabs facing toward the center. Place the circle in the center of the ring on top of the tabs to form a bottom. Tape the tabs to the bottom of the circle.

5. Put a thumbtack through the center hole of the base and attach it to a plastic lid or cup.

6. Cut and tape the other strips A to A and B to B. Select an image strip and put it along the inside circumference and below the slots in the drum.

**BOTTOM
OF
ZOETROPE**

EXAMINATION OF THE LARYNX SINGULAR PUBLISHING GROUP SAN DIEGO CALIFORNIA

STROBOSCOPIC EXAMINATION OF THE LARYNX SINGULAR PUBLISHING GROUP SAN DIEGO CALIFORNIA

VIDEO STROBOSCOPIC EXAMINATION OF THE LARYNX SINGULAR PUBLISHING GROUP SAN DIEGO CALIFORNIA

MHIRANO AND dBLESS VIDEO STROBOSCOPIC EXAMINATION OF THE LARYNX SINGULAR PUBLISHING GROUP SAN DIEGO CALIFORNIA

MHIRANO AND dBLESS VIDEOSTROBOSCOPIC

MHIRANO AND dBLESS

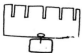

7. With the zoetrope at eye level, spin it while looking through the slots to observe vocal fold movement illustrating points made in this book.

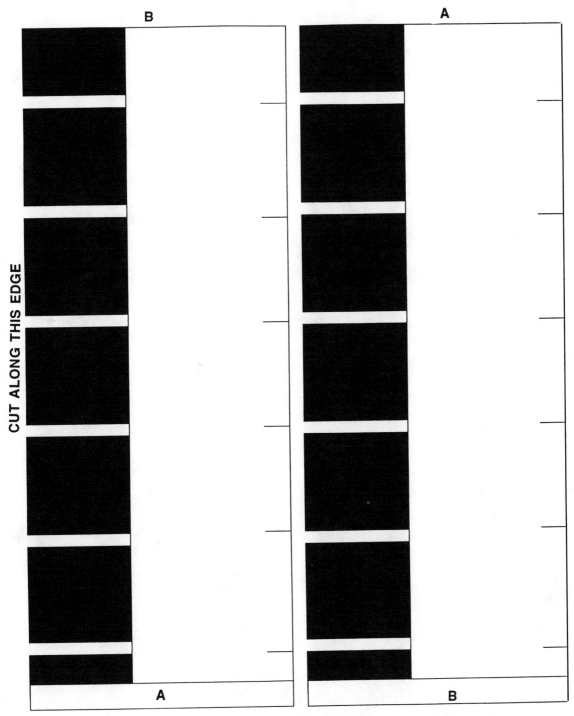

CUT ALONG THIS EDGE

B

A

A

B

SIDES OF ZOETROPE

211

CUT ALONG THIS EDGE

B

A

B

A

A

B

A

B

IMAGE STRIP 1a   **IMAGE SRIP 1b**   **IMAGE STRIP 2a**   **IMAGE STRIP 2b**

213

CUT ALONG THIS EDGE

B

A

B

A

IMAGE STRIP 3a **IMAGE STRIP 3b** **IMAGE STRIP 4a** **IMAGE STRIP 4b**

A

B

A

B

215

References

Alberti, P. W. (1978). The diagnostic role of laryngeal stroboscopy. Symposium on advances in otolaryngologic diagnosis. *Otolaryngologic Clinics of North America, 11,* 347–354.

American Speech-Language-Hearing Association (1990). AIDS/HIV Update. *ASHA, 32.*

American Speech-Language-Hearing Association Ad Hoc Committee on Advances in Clinical Practice. (1992a). Vocal tract visualization and imaging. *ASHA, 34,* 37–40.

American Speech-Language-Hearing Association Ad Hoc Committee on Advances in Clinical Practice. (1992b). Sedation and topical anesthetics in audiology and speech-language pathology. *ASHA, 34,* 41–42.

Andrews, A. H., Jr., & Gould, W. J. (1977). Laryngeal and nasopharyngeal indirect telescope. *Annals of Otology, Rhinology, and Laryngology, 86,* 627.

Baken, J. R. (1987). *Clinical measurement of speech and voice.* Boston: College-Hill Press.

Bastian, R. W. (1987). Laryngeal image biofeedback for voice disorder patients. *Journal of Voice, 1,* 279–282.

Beck, J., & Schönharl, E. (1954). Ein neues mikrophongesteuertes Lichtblitz-Stroboskop. *HNO (Berlin), 4,* 449–452.

Bless, D. M. (1988). Voice disorders in the adult: Assessment. In D. E. Yoder & R. Kent (Eds.), *Decision making in speech-language pathology* (pp. 136–139). Philadelphia: B. C. Decker.

Bless, D. M., & Hirano, M. (1982, November). *Estimation of glottal airflow and maximum phonation time as a clinical tool.* Presentation at the American Speech-Language-Hearing Association Annual Convention, Toronto, Ontario, Canada.

Bless, D. M., Hirano, M., & Feder, R. (1984). Stroboscopic evaluation of the larynx workshop, Madison, WI.

Booth, J. R., & Childers, D.G. (1979). Automated analysis of ultra high-speed laryngeal films. *IEEE Transactions on Biomedical Engineering, 4,* 185–192.

Boves, L. (1984). *The phonetic basis of perceptual ratings of running speech.* Cinnaminson, NJ: Foris.

Brüel & Kjaer Co. (1984) *Rhino-larynx Stroboscope, Type 4914.* Marlborough, MA: Brüel & Kjaer.

Cantarella, G. (1987). Value of flexible videolaryngoscopy in the study of laryngeal morphology and functions. *Journal of Voice, 1,* 353–358.

Casper, J. K., Brewer, D. W., & Colton, R. H. (1987). Pitfalls and problems in flexible fiberoptic videolaryngoscopy. *Journal of Voice, 1,* 347–352.

Centers for Disease Control. (1988, June). Perspectives in disease prevention and health promotion. *Morbidity and Mortality Weekly Report, 37,* 377–388.

Childers, D. G. (1977). Laryngeal pathology detection. *Critical Reviews in Bioengineering, 2,* 375–426.

Colman, M. F., & Reynolds, R. (1985). The use of topical cocaine to prevent laryngospasm after general anesthesia on endoscopy procedures, *Laryngoscope, 95,* 474.

Colton, R. H. (1972). Phonational range in the modal and falsetto registers. *Journal of Speech and Hearing Research, 15,* 708–713.

Colton, R. H., & Casper, J. K. (1990). *Understanding voice problems: A physiological perspective for diagnosis and treatment.* Baltimore: Williams & Wilkins.

Colton, R. H., Casper, J. K., Brewer, D. W., & Conture, E. G. (1989). Digital processing of laryngeal images: A preliminary report. *Journal of Voice, 3,* 132–142.

Colton, R., Casper, J., Brewer, D., Woo, P., & Bless, D.M. (1991). *Stroboscopic evaluation of the larynx.* Workshop. American Speech-Language-Hearing Association, Annual Convention, Atlanta, GA.

Conture, E. G., Schwartz, H., & Brewer, D. W. (1986). Laryngeal behavior during stuttering: A further study. *Journal of Speech and Hearing Research, 28,* 233–240.

Davidson, T. M., Bone, R. C., & Nahum, A. M. (1974). Flexible fiberoptic laryngobronchoscopy. *Laryngoscope, 84,* 1876–1882.

Dellon, A. L., Clifford, A. H., & Chretien, D. B. (1975). Fiberoptic endoscopy in the head and neck region. *Plastic and Reconstructive Surgery, 55,* 466–471.

Edgerton, H. E. (1970). *Electronic flash strobe.* New York: McGraw-Hill.

Evers, W., Racz, G. B. Glazer, J., & Dubkin, A. B. (1967). Orahesive as a protection for the teeth during general anaesthesia and endoscopy. *Canadian Anaesthetists Society Journal, 14,* 123–128.

Faure, M. A., & Muller, A. (1992). Stroboscopy [Special Article]. *Journal of Voice, 6,* 139–148.

Fex, S., & Elmqvist, D. (1973). Endemic recurrent laryngeal nerve paresis. Correlation between EMG and stroboscopic findings. *Acta Otolaryngologica, 75,* 368–369.

Fujita, H., & Fujita, T. (1981). *Textbook of histology, Part 1.* Tokyo: Igaku Shoin.

Garcia, M. (1855). Observations of the human voice. *Philosophical Magainze Journal of Science, 10,* 511–513.

Gottfried, E. L. (1992). Voice tests and lab tests. *Voice and Voice Disorders 3, American Speech and Hearing Association Newsletter, 2,* 1–3.

Gould, W. J., Kojima, H., & Lambiase, A. (1979). A technique for stroboscopic examination of the vocal folds using fiberoptics. *Archives of Otolaryngology, 105,* 285.

Groening, M. (1991). *The Simpsons fun book.* New York: Matt Groening Productions, Inc., HarperCollins.

Harley, B. (1988). *Optical toys.* Princes Risborough, UK: Shire Publications, Ltd.

Helmholtz, H. (1948). *Sensations of tone* (6th ed., pp. 88–102). New York: Peter Smith.

Hibi, S. R., Bless, D. M., Hirano, M., & Yoshida, T. (1988). Distortions of videofiberoscopy imaging: Reconsideration and correction. *Journal of Voice, 2,* 168–175.

Hirano, M. (1974). Morphological structure of the vocal cord as a vibrator and its variations. *Folia Phoniatrica, 26,* 89–94.

Hirano, M. (1981a). *Clinical examination of voice.* New York: Springer-Verlag.

Hirano, M. (1981b). Structure of the vocal fold in normal and diseased states: Anatomical and physical study. In *Proceedings of the Conference on the Assessment of Vocal Pathology, American Speech and Hearing Association Report, 11,* 69.

Hirano, M. (1988). Endolaryngeal microsurgery. In G. M. English (Ed.), *Otolaryngology* (Vol. 3, pp. 1–22). Philadelphia: J. B. Lippincott.

Hirano, M., Matsushita, H., Kawasaki, H., Yoshida, Y., & Koike, Y. (1974). Vibration of the vocal cords with unilateral polyp. An ultra high speed cinematographic study. *Journal of Otolaryngology of Japan, 77,* 593–610.

Hirano, M., Vennard, W., & Ohala, J. (1970) Regulation of register, pitch, and intensity of voice: An electromyographic investigation of intrinsic laryngeal muscles. *Folia Phoniatrica, 22,* 1–20.

Hirano, M., Yoshida, Y., Yoshida, T., & Tateishi, O. (1987). Strobofiberscopic video recording of vocal fold vibration. *Annals of Otology, Rhinology, and Laryngology, 91,* 354–358.

Hirose, H. (1988). High-speed digital imaging of vocal fold vibration. *Acta Oto-laryngologica (Stockholm), 458,* 151–153.

Hiroto, I. (1966). The mechanism of phonation, its pathophysiologic aspects. *Oto Rhino Laryngology Clinic, Kyoto, 59,* 229–291.

Holmberg, E., & Leanderson, R. (1983). Laryngeal aerodynamics and voice quality. In V. Lawrence (Ed.), *Transcripts of the Eleventh Symposium on Care of the Professional Voice, Part II, Medical/Surgical Sessions: Papers.* New York: The Voice Foundation.

International Association of Logopedics and Phoniatrics (IALP) Voice Committee. (1992). Discussion of assessment topics. *Journal of Voice, 6,* 194–210.

Isshiki, N., & Ringel, R. L. (1964) Airflow during the production of selected consonants. *Journal of Speech and Hearing Research, 7,* 151–164.

Iwata, S. (1988). Aerodynamic aspects for phonation in normal and pathologic larynges. In O. Fujimura (Ed.), *Vocal physiology: Voice production, mechanics and functions.* New York: Raven Press.

Jephcott, A. (1984). The Macintosh Laryngoscope: A historical note on its clinical and commercial development. *Anaesthesia, 39,* 474–479.

Karnell, M. P. (1989). Synchronized videostroboscopy and electroglottography. *Journal of Voice, 3,* 68–75.

Karnell, M. P. (1991). Laryngeal perturbation analysis: Minimum length of analysis window. *Journal of Speech and Hearing Research, 34,* 544–548.

Kitajima, K. (1985). Airflow study of pathologic larynges using a hotwired flowmeter. *Annals of Otology, Rhinology, and Laryngology, 94,* 195–197.

Kivenson, G. (1965). *Industrial stroboscopy.* New York: Hayden Book Company.

Konrad, H. R., Hople, D. M., & Bussen, J. (1981). Use of strobofiberscopic video recording of vocal fold vibration. *Annals of Otology, Rhinology, and Laryngology, 90,* 398–400.

Ladefoged, P., & McKinney, N. P. (1963). Loudness, sound pressure, and subglottic pressure in speech. *Journal of the Acoustical Society of America, 35,* 454–460.

Laver, J., Hiller, S., & Mackenzie, J. (1992). Acoustic waveform perturbations and voice disorders. *Journal of Voice, 6,* 115–126.

Linville, S. E., & Fisher, H. (1985). Acoustic characteristics of perceived versus actual aging. Controlled phonation by adult females. *Journal of the Acoustical Society of America, 78,* 40–48.

Lofqvist, A., Carlborg, B., & Kitzing, P. (1982) Initial validation of an indirect measure of subglottal pressure during vowels. *Journal of the Acoustical Society of America, 72,* 633–635.

Lopez, S. (1989). Patient variable biases in clinical judgment: Conceptual overview and methodological considerations. *Psychological Bulletin, 106,* 184–203.

Luchsinger, R., & Arnold, G. E. (1965). *Voice-speech-language* (2nd ed.). (G. E. Arnold & E. R. Finkbeiner, Trans.) Belmont, CA: Wadsworth.

Ludlow, C., (1981). Research needs for the assessment of phonatory function. In C. Ludlow & M. Hart (Eds.), *Proceedings of the Conference on the Assessment of Vocal Pathology* (pp. 3–8). Danville, IL: American Speech-Language-Hearing Association.

McKelvie, P., Grey, P., & North, C. (1970). Laryngeal strobomicroscope. *Lancet, 2,* 503–504.

Moore D. M., & von Leden, H. (1958). Dynamic variations of the vibratory pattern in the normal larynx. *Folia Phoniatrica, 10,* 205–238.

Mysak, E. D. (1959). Pitch and duration characteristics of older males. *Journal of Speech and Hearing Research, 2,* 46–54.

National Institute for Deafness and Other Communication Disorders. (1990, September). Assessment of speech and voice production: Research and clinical applications. *Monograph, Proceedings of a Conference,* Bethesda, MD.

Oertel, M. J. (1895). Das Laryngo-Stroboskop und die laryngostroboskopische Untersuchung. *Archivs für Laryngologie und Rhinologie, 3,* 1–5.

Orlikoff, R. F., & Baken, R. J. (1990) Consideration of the relationship between the fundamental frequency of phonation and vocal jitter. *Folia Phoniatrica, 42,* 31–40.

Peppard, R. C., & Bless, D. M. (1989). Does topical anesthetic affect videostroboscopic examination of the larynx? *ASHA, 31,* 86.

Peppard, R., Bless, D. M., & Milenkovic, P. (1988). Comparison of young adult singers and nonsingers with vocal nodules. *Journal of Voice, 2,* 250–260.

Raj, P. P., Forestner, J., Watson, T. D., Morris, R. E., & Jenkins, M. T. (1974). Techniques for fiberoptic laryngoscopy in anaesthesia. *Anaesthesia and Analgesia, 53,* 708–714.

Ramig, L. (1975). *Examiner bias in perceptual ratings of nasality in cleft palate speakers.* Unpublished master's thesis, University of Wisconsin, Madison.

Rammage, L. A., Peppard, R. C., & Bless, D. M. (1992). Aerodynamic, laryngoscopic, and perceptual acoustic characteristics in dysphonic females with posterior glottal chinks: A retrospective study. *Journal of Voice, 6,* 64–78.

Rothenberg, M. (1973). A new inverse-filtering technique for deriving the glottal airflow during waveform during voicing. *Journal of the Acoustical Society of America, 53,* 1632–1645.

Saito, S., Fukuda, H., Kitahara, S., & Isogai, Y. (1984). Curved laryngotelescope. *Laryngoscope, 94,* 1103–1105.

Saito, S., Isogai, Y., & Fukuda, H. (1981). A newly developed laryngotelescope. *Journal of the Japanese Bronchesophagological Society, 32,* 328–331.

Sawashima, M., Totsuka, G., Kobayashi, T., & Hirose, M. (1968). Reconstructive surgery for hoarseness due to unilateral vocal cord paralysis. *Archives of Otolaryngology, 87,* 289.

Shearer, W. M. (1984). Academic and instructional applications for microcomputers. In A. H. Schwartz (Ed.), *The handbook of microcomputer applications in communication disorders* (pp. 193–218). San Diego: College-Hill Press.

Scherer, R. C., Gould, W. J., Titze, I. R., Meyers, A. D., & Sataloff, R. T. (1988). Preliminary evaluation of selected acoustic and glottographic measures for clinical phonatory function analysis. *Journal of Voice, 2,* 230–244.

Schönharl, E. (1960a). *Die Stroboskopie in der praktischen Laryngologie.* Stuttgart: Georg Thieme Verlag.

Schönharl, E. (1960b). Zur stroboskopischen diagnostik von stimmbandkarzinom und tuberkulose. *Aktuelle Probleme der Phoniatrie und Logapaedie, 1,* 118–124.

Selkin, S. G. (1983a). Flexible fiberoptics for laryngeal photography. *Laryngoscope, 93,* 657–658.

Selkin, S. G. (1983b). The otolaryngologist and flexible fiberoptics: Photographic consideration. *Journal of Otolaryngology, 12,* 223–227.

Sercarz, J. A., Berke, G. S., Gerratt, B. R., Kreiman, J., Ming, Y., & Navidad, M. (1992). Synchronizing videostroboscopic images of human laryngeal vibration with physiological signals. *American Journal of Otolaryngology, 13,* 40–44.

Sercarz, J. A., Berke, G. S., Ming, Y., Gerratt, B. R., & Navidad, M. (1992). Videostroboscopy of human vocal fold paralysis. *Annals of Otology, Rhinology, and Laryngology, 101,* 567–577.

Shipp, T. (1973). Intra-oral air pressure and lip occlusion in midvocalic stop consonant production. *Journal of Phonetics, 1,* 167–170.

Silberman, H. D., Wilf, H., & Tucker, J. A. (1967). Flexible fiberoptic nasopharyngolaryngoscope. *Annals of Oto-Rhino-Laryngology, 85,* 640–645.

Smitheran, J., & Hixon, T. (1971). A clinical method for

estimating laryngeal airway resistance during vowel production. *Journal of Speech and Hearing Disorders, 46,* 138–146.

Stoicheff, M. (1981). Speaking fundamental frequency characteristics of nonsmoking female adults. *Journal of Speech and Hearing Research, 24,* 437–441.

Stone, R. E., Jr., & Lingeman, R. E. (1987). *A proposal for insurance coverage of laryngeal videoendoscopic and videostroboscopic examinations.* Unpublished manuscript, Indiana University School of Medicine, Department of Otolaryngology-Head and Neck Surgery, Indianapolis.

Suzuki, Y., Saito, S., Hayasaki, H., & Murakami, Y. (1964). *Société Francaise d'Oto-Rhino-Laryngologie et de Pathologie Cervico-Faciale, 67,* 752.

Teitler, N. (1992). *Examiner bias: Influence of patient history on perceptual ratings of videostroboscopy.* Unpublished master's thesis, University of Wisconsin-Madison.

Timcke, R. (1956a). Die Synchron-stroboskopie von menschlichen Stimmlippen bzw. ähnlichen Schallquellen und Messung der öffungszeit. *Zeitschrift für Laryngologie und Rhinologie, 35,* 331–335.

Timcke, R. (1956b). Laryngostroboskopie mittels eines neuartigen synchronstroboskops. *Zeitschrift fur Hals-, Nasen- und Kehlkopfheilkunde, 169,* 539–543.

Titze, I. (1988). The physics of small-amplitude oscillation of the vocal folds. *Journal of the Acoustical Society of America, 83,* 1536–1552.

Titze, I. (1989). Physiologic and acoustic differences between male and female voices. *Journal of the Acoustical Society of America, 85,* 1699–1707.

Titze, I., & Sundberg, J. (1992). Vocal intensity in speech and singing. *Journal of the Acoustical Society of America, 91,* 2936–2946.

Tobin, H. A. (1980). Office fiberoptic laryngeal photography. *Otolaryngology-Head Neck Surgery, 88,* 172–173.

von Leden, H. V., Moore, P., & Timcke, R. (1960). Laryngeal vibrations: III. The pathologic larynx. *Archives of Otology, 71,* 1232–1250.

Weismer, G. (1984). Acoustic analysis of dysarthric speech: Perceptual correlates and physiological inferences. In J. C. Rosenbeck (Ed.), *Seminars in Speech, Hearing and Language, 5,* 293–314.

Wendler, J. (1992). Stroboscopy [Special Article]. *Journal of Voice, 6,* 149–154.

White, J. F., & Knight, R. E. (1984). Office videofiberoptic laryngoscopy. *Laryngoscope, 94,* 1166–1169.

Williams, G. T., Farquharson, I. M., & Anthony, J. K. (1975). Fiberoptic laryngoscopy in the assessment of laryngeal disorders. *Journal of Laryngology and Otology, 89,* 299–316.

Wilson, F. B., Kudryk, W. H., & Sych, A. (1986). The development of flexible fiberoptic video nasendoscopy (FFVN): Clinical, teaching, research applications. *ASHA, 28,* 25–30.

Wilson, F., & Star, C. (1985). Use of the phonation analyzer as a clinical tool. *Journal of Speech and Hearing Disorders, 50,* 351–356.

Yanagihara, N. (1967). Significance of harmonic changes and noise components in hoarseness. *Journal of Speech and Hearing Research, 10,* 531–541.

Yanagisawa, E., Owens, T. W., Strothers, G., & Honda, K. (1983). Videolaryngoscopy: A comparison of fiberscopic and telescopic documentation. *Annals of Otology, Rhinology, and Laryngology, 92,* 430–436.

Yoshida, Y. (1977). An improved model of laryngostroboscope. *Otolaryngology, 49,* 663–669.

Bibliography

OVERVIEW OF STROBOSCOPY APPLIED TO LARYNGEAL IMAGING

Abitbol, J., LeHuche, F., & Chevrie-Muller, C. (1975). Exploration dynamique. À propos de 500 EDV. *Bulletin d'Audiophonologie (Besançon)*, 17, 60–69.

Alberti, P. W. (1978). The diagnostic role of laryngeal stroboscopy. Symposium on advances in otolaryngologic diagnosis. *Otolaryngologic Clinics of North America*, 11, 347–354.

Allessi, D. M., & von Leden, H. (1992). Stroboscopy and phonosurgery. [A letter to the editor]. *Archives of Otolaryngology and Head and Neck Surgery*, 118, 1003–1004.

Arndt, H. J. (1986). Stroboskopische Diagnostik. *Sprache-Stimme-Gehör (Stuttgart)*, 10, 81–82.

Baken, J. R. (1987). *Clinical measurement of speech and voice*. Boston: College-Hill Press.

Barth, V. (1977). Die Lupenstroboskopie. *HNO*, 25, 35.

Barth, V. (1982). Die Lupenstroboskopie als Möglichkeit der Funkdiagnostik von Stimmstörungen und Stimmlippenprozessen (p. 28). Knittlingen: R. Wolf GmbH.

Barth, V., & Pilorget, J. (1983). La stroboscopie laryngée. *Revue de Laryngologie d'Otologie et de Rhinologie (Bordeaux)*, 104, 359–364.

Barth, V., & Schatzle, W. (1981). Fünf Jahre klinische Erfahrung mit der Lupenstroboskopie. *Sprache-Stimme-Gehör (Stuttgart)*, 5, 3–5.

Bastian, R. W. (1987a). Laryngeal image biofeedback for voice disorder patients. *Journal of Voice*, 1, 279–282.

Bastian, R. W. (1987b). Laryngeal videostroboscopy and photography for the diagnosis and management of voice disorders. *Insights in Otolaryngology*, 2.

Beck, J., & Schonharl, E. (1954). Ein neues mikrophongesteuertes Lichtblitz-Stroboskop. *HNO (Berlin)*, 4, 449–452.

Bekbulatov, G. T. (1969). Stroboskopiia votsenke funksional'nugo vosstabivkeniia golosovogo apparata posle operatsii na golosovvykh sladkakh. *Vestnik Oto-rinolaringologii (Moskva)*, 31, 52–54.

Bless, D. M. (1984). *Stroboscopic evaluation of the larynx*. Unpublished handout (p. 31). University of Wisconsin-Madison.

Bless, D. M., Hirano, M., & Feder, R. (1987). Videostroboscopic examination of the larynx. *Ear, Nose, and Throat Journal, Special Issue*, 66, 289–296.

Bohme G. (1965). Die Wirksamkeit der Elektrotherapie bei Kehlkopferkränkungen im stroboskopischen Bild. *Laryngologie*, 481–488.

Bohme, G. (1974). Stroboskopische für Diagnostik bei Kehlkopfkarzinom. *Materia Medica Nordmark*, 26, 86–95.

Brüel & Kjaer Co. (1984). *Rino-larynx Stroboscope, Type 4914*. Marlborough, MA: Brüel & Kjaer.

Chaplin, V. L., & Iakovleva, I. I. (1964). Stroboskopiia detei kapelly mal'chikov. *Novosti Meditsinskoi Tekhniki*, 2, 41–44.

Colton, R. H., & Casper, J. K. (1990). *Understanding voice problems: A physiological perspective for diagnosis and treatment*. Baltimore: Williams & Wilkins.

Cornut, G., & Bouchayer, M. (1972). Indications phoniatriques de la microchirurgie laryngée. *Journal Français d'Oto Rhino Laryngologie Audiophonologie et Chirurgie Maxillo-Faciale*, 22, 5–52

Cornut, G., & Bouchayer, M. (1973). Apport de la microchirurgie laryngée dans le traitement du nodule de la corde vocale. *Folia Phoniatrica*, 24, 431–437.

Cornut, G., & Bouchayer, M. (1977a). Indications phoniatriques et resultats fonctionnels de la microchirurgie laryngée. *Bulletin d'Audiophonologie*, 7, 5–52.

Cornut, G., & Bouchayer, M. (1977b). Voix et microchirurgie laryngée. *Bulletin d' Audiophonologie*, 7, 5–51.

Cornut, G., & Bouchayer, M. (1985). Les therapeutiques phoniatriques de la voix chantée. *Revue de Laryngologie, Otologie, Rhinologie (Bordeaux)*, 106, 289–294.

Cornut, G., & Bouchayer, M. (1988b). *Medical instrumentation: Video stroboscopy. Assessment of cases for phonosurgery* (p. 6). Stockholm: Brüel & Kjaer.

Cornut, G., & Lafon, J. C. (1960). Vibrations neuromusculaires des cordes vocales et theories de la phonation. *Journal Français d'Oto Rhino Laryngologie Audiophonologie et Chirurgie Maxillo-Faciale, 9,* 317–324.

Costamagna, D. (1988). *La vidéo-stroboscopie en laryngologie* (Vol. 2, 2nd ed, pp. 132, 230). Nice, France: Thése Médicine.

Costamagna, D. (1990). La vidéo-laryngostroboscopie. *Bulletin d'Audiophonologie, 6,* 491–546.

Croft, T. A. (1971). Failure of visual estimation of motion under strobe. *Nature, 231,* 397.

Damste, H. (1957). Stroboscopic fixation of the vocal cords. *Practica Oto-Rhino-Laryngologica, 19,* 438

Damste, H., & Huizinga, E. (1959). *Practica Oto-Rhino-Laryngologica, 21,* 349.

Darasovenau, C., & Popoviciu, L. (1968). *Ceskoslovenska Otolaryngologie (Praha), 16,* 285.

Edgerton, H. E. (1970). *Electronic flash, strobe.* New York: McGraw-Hill.

Ernst, T. (1959). The stroboscopic recognition of functional voice disorders by means of singing and speaking stress. *Archiv für Ohren- Nasen- und Kehlkopfheilkunde, 175,* 452–455.

Ernst, R. (1960). Stroboscopic studies in professional speakers. *HNO, 8,* 170–174.

Faure, M. A., & Muller, A. (1992). Stroboscopy [Special Article]. *Journal of Voice, 6,* 139–148.

Fenton, E., Niimi, S., Harris, K. S., & Sehley, W. S. (1976, November). *Stroboscopic investigations of larynges of Parkinson's disease patients.* Paper presented at the American Speech and Hearing Association Annual Convention.

Fex, S. (1970). Judging the movements of vocal cords in larynx paralysis. *Acta Oto-laryngologica (Stockholm), 263,* 82–83.

Fex, S., & Elmqvist, D. (1973). Endemic recurrent laryngeal nerve patesis correlation between EMG and stroboscopic findings. *Acta-Oto-Laryngologica, 75,* 368–369.

Frêche, C., DeJean, Y., DeMard, F. (1984). *La voix humaine et ses troubles, 1ère éd.* (p. 286). Paris: Societé Française d'Oto Rhino Laryngologie.

Frint, T. (1974). Experimentelle Untersuchungen seltener stimmphänomene bei einem Fall von spastischer Dysphonie. *Folia Phoniatrica, 26,* 422–427.

Frint, T., & Kelemen, A. (1969). Inspiratorische Stimmbildung psychogenen Ursprunges. *Folia Phoniatrica, 21,* 105–111.

Fulgencio, M. S. (1978) Laryngeal stroboscopy. *AMB, 24,* 17–18.

Gall, V. (1984). Strip kymography of the glottis. *Archives of Oto- Rhino- Laryngology, 240,* 287–293.

Gallivan, G. J., Dawson, J. A, & Opfell, A. P. (1990). Videolaryngoscopy after endotracheal intubation: Part II. A critical care perspective of lesions affecting voice. *Journal of Voice, 4,* 159–164.

Gelfer, P. M., & Bultemeyer, D. K. (1990). Evaluation of vocal fold vibratory patterns in normal voices. *Journal of Voice, 4,* 335–345.

Gerull, G., Gesen, M., Mrowinski, D., & Rudolph, N. (1972). Laryngeal stroboscopy using a scanning microphone. *HNO 20,* 369.

Gould, W. J., Kojima, H., & Lambaise, A. (1979). A technique for stroboscopic examination of the vocal folds using fiberoptics. *Archives of Otolaryngology, 105,* 285.

Greiner, G. F., Dillenschneider, E., & Conraux, C. (1968). Stroboscopic and sonographic aspects of the traumatic larynx. *Journal Français d'Oto Rhino Laryngologie, d'Audiophonologie et Chirurgie Maxillo-Faciale, 17,* 237–241.

Grey, P. (1973). Microlaryngostroboscopy and singer's nodes. *Journal of the Otolaryngological Society of Australia, 3,* 525–527.

Haas, E. (1974). Heiserkeit und Kehlkopfkrebs. *Therapiewoche, 24,* 5632–5682.

Haas, E., & Bildstein, P. (1974). Die Bedeutung der Stroboskopie für die Früerkennung des Stimmlippenkrebses. *Zeitschrift für Laryngologie, Rhinologie, Otolaryngologie, und ihre Grenzgebiete, 53,* 169–172.

Hala, B., & Honnty, L. (1931). Cinematography of vocal cords by means of stroboscope and great speed. *Otolaryngologia Slavica, 3,* 1–12.

Halbedl, G. (1964). Grundlagen der technik der Kehlfopfstroboskopie. In *Handbuch Medizin Elektronik, Teil II.* Berlin: VEB Technik.

Harley, B. (1988). *Optical toys.* Princes Risborough, UK: Shire Publications, Ltd.

Hartmann, H. G. (1985). *Diagnosis using stroboscopy.* Naerum, Denmark: Brüel et Kjaer.

Heinemann, M. (1969). Klinische Untersuchungen beim sulcus glottidis. *Zeitschrift für Laryngologie und Rhinologie, 48(11),* 801–807.

Hirano, M. (1981). *Clinical examination of voice.* New York: Springer-Verlag.

Hirano, M., Gould, W. J., Lambiase, A., & Kakita, Y. (1981). Vibratory behavior of the vocal folds in a case with a unilateral polyp. *Folia Phoniatrica, 33,* 275–284.

Hirano, M., & Hartmann, H. G. (1986). Aspects of videostroboscopy in practice. In *Proceedings of the 20th IALP Congress* (p. 402). Tokyo: The Organizing Committee of the XXth Congress of the International Association of Logopedics and Phoniatrics.

Hirano, M., Nozoe, I., Shin, T., & Maeyama, T. (1972). Vibration of the vocal cords with recurrent laryngeal nerve palsy. A stroboscopic investigation. *Practica Oto Rhino Laryngologica, 65,* 1037–1047.

Hirano, M., Yoshida, Y., Yoshida, T., & Tateishi, O. (1985). Strobofiberscopic video recording of vocal fold vibration. *Annals of Otology, Rhinology and Laryngology, 94,* 588–590.

Hirano, M., Yoshida, Y., Yoshida, T., & Tateishi, O. (1987). Strobofiberscopic video recording of vocal fold vibration. *Annals of Otology, Rhinology and Laryngology, 91,* 354–358.

Hollien, H., Coleman, R., & Moore, P. (1968). Stroboscopic laminagraphy of the larynx during phonation. *Acta Oto-laryngologica (Stockholm), 65,* 209-251.

Husson, R. (1951). Stroboscopic study of reflex modifications of vibration of vocal cords produced by experimental stimulations of auditory and trigeminal nerves. *Comptes Rendus de l' Academie Science, Paris, 232,* 1247–1249.

Husson, R. (1980). Principal facts of vocal physiology and pathology gained by laryngostroboscopy. *Reviews of Laryngology Otology and Rhinology, 57,* 1132–1145.

Ishikawa, T. (1983). Clinical investigation of vocal cord paralysis. *Practica Otologica Kyoto, 76,* 747–752.

Izdebski, K., Ross, J. C., & Klein, J. C. (1990). Transoral rigid laryngovideostroboscopy (phonoscopy). *Seminars in Speech and Language, 1,* 16–26.

Kallen, L. A. (1932). Laryngostroboscopy in the practice of otolaryngology. *Archives of Otolaryngology, 16,* 791–807.

Kallen, L. A., & Polin, H. S. (1934). A physiological Stroboscope. *Science, 80,* 592.

Kallen, L. A., & Polin, H. S. (1937). Ein physiologisches stroboskop. *Monatsschrift für Ohrenheilkunde und Laryngo-Rhinologie, 71,* 1177–1181.

Karnell, M. P. (1989). Synchronized videostroboscopy and electroglottography. *Journal of Voice, 3,* 68–75.

Kirikae, I. (1943). Über den Bewegungsvorgang an den Stimmlippen und die Öffnungs- und verschlubzeit der Stimmritze während der Phonation. *Journal of Otolaryngology (Japan), 49,* 236–262.

Kitajima, K. (1985). Airflow studies of pathologic larynges using a tjaPage 248 owmeter. *Annals of Otology, Rhinology, and Laryngology, 94,* 195–197.

Kittel, G. (1977). *Farb-Video-Stroboskopie.* Demonstration, 52 Jahrestag. Deutsch Gestalt Sprach- und Stimmheilkunde, Bad Reichenhall, Germany.

Kittel, G. (1978). Lupens-Mikro-TV-Farbstroboskopie mit Amplituden-bestimmungsmöglichkeiten. *HNO, 26,* 94–96.

Kitzing, P. (1985). Stroboscopy — A pertinent laryngological examination. *Otolaryngology (London), 14,* 151–175.

Kleinsasser, O. (1968). *Microlaringoscopia y microcinurgia endolaringea.* Barcelona, Spain: Cientifico-Medica.

Kmucha, S. T., Yanagisawa, E., & Estill, J. (1990). Endolaryngeal changes during high-intensity phonation. Videolaryngoscopic observations. *Journal of Voice, 4,* 346–354.

Koeppen, K. (1988). *Quantitativ Untersuchungen zur klinischen Wertigkeit stroboskopischer Befunde.* Medizinische Dissertation A, Berlin.

Koike, Y. (1987, January). *Quantitative measures of stroboscopic images of the larynx.* Paper presented at the Fifth Vocal Fold Physiology Conference, Tokyo.

Koike, Y., Daito, N., & Imaizumi, S. (1987). Analisis cuantitativo de las vibraciones de los replieques vocales mediante cine-estroboscopia. *Revista Logopaedica Foniatria Audiologica, 7,* 126–130.

Konrad, H. R., Hople, D. M., & Bussen, J. (1981). Use of strobofiberscopic video recording of vocal fold vibration. *Annals of Otology, Rhinology, and Laryngology, 90,* 398–400.

Krahulee, I. (1970). Importance of stroboscopy in laryngology. *Ceskoslovenska Otolaryngologica, 19,* 29–31.

Krahulec, I., Skrovanek, S., & Kostolansky, P. (1970). Sound meter for assessing the intensity of the voice in stroboscopic examinations. *Ceskoslovenska Otolaryngologica, 19,* 44–46.

Kristensen, H. K., & Zilstorff-Pederson, K. (1982). Synchrono-electro-stroboscopie examination of the vocal cords. *Nordisk Medicin, 68,* 927–929.

Kruse, E. (1988). Stroboscopic diagnosis and differential diagnosis of organically caused dysphonia. In *Proceedings of the 15th Union of European Phoniatricians Congress* (Erlangen), Köln: Deutscher Artze Verlag.

Lehman, J. J., Bless, D. M., & Brandenburg, J. H. (1988). An objective assessment of voice production after radiation therapy for stage I squamous cell carcinoma of the glottis. *Otolaryngology-Head and Neck Surgery, 98,* 121–129.

Leito, F. B., Morganti, A. P., Elisabetscky, M., & Mantoanelli, J. B. (1968). Stroboscopy control of phonetic sound before and after tracheal intubation. *Revista Brasileira de Anestesiologia, 18,* 182–191.

Loebell, H. (1926). A new stroboscope for examining vibrations of vocal cord. *Zeitschrift für Hals, Nasen und Ohrenheilkunde, 15,* 371.

Luchsinger, R. (1943). Die Elektrostroboskopie und harmonische Vibration mittelst eines Tongenerators. *Schweizerische Medizinische Wochenschrift, 73,* 135–136.

Luchsinger, R. (1948). Stroboscopic symptomatology. *Practica Oto-Rhino-Laryngologica, 10,* 209–214.

MacKay, D. M. (1970). Fragmentation of binocular vision in stroboscopic illumination. *Nature, 227,* 518.

Maliutin, E. M. (1980). Stroboscopic phenomena in vocal students. *Russkaia Klinika, 13,* 681–691.

Marcos, J., & Pedrosa, C. Revista media del hospital general. *Asturias, 4,* 14.

Mareev, V. M., & Papshitsckii, Y. A. (1971). Stroboscopy in hyperplastic and tumor processes of the larynx. *Oto-rhinolaryngology, 33,* 10–12.

Mareev, V. M., & Papshitsckii, Y. A. (1973). Stroboskopiia pri giperplasticheskikh i opukhdevykh protessakh gortani. *Versnik Oto-rino-laryngologii (Moskva), 76,* 495–500.

Matsushita, H. (1975). The vibratory mode of the vocal folds in the excised larynx. *Folia Phonatrica, 27,* 7–18.

McKelvie, W. B. (1944). Stroboscope using grid-controlled tube, "strobotron." *Journal of Laryngology and Otology (London), 59,* 464–465.

McKelvie, P., Grey, P., & North, C. (1970). Laryngeal stroboscope. *Lancet, 2,* 503–504.

Merriman, J. S. (1977). Stroboscopic photography as a research instrument. *Research Quarterly of the American Association of Health and Physical Education, 48,* 628–631.

Milutinovic, Z. (1990). Advantages of indirect videostroboscopic surgery of the larynx. *Folia Phoniatrica, 42,* 77–82.

Minnigerode, B. (1967). The defiguration phenomenon in motion perception and its effect on stroboscopic laryngoscopy. *Laryngologie Rhinologie und Otologie, 101,* 33–38.

Monday, L. A., Bouchayer, M., Cornut, G., & Roch, J. B. (1983). Epidermoid cysts of the vocal cords. *Annals of Otology, Rhinology, and Laryngology, 92,* 124–127.

Monday, L. A., Bouchayer, M., Roch, J. B., & Loire, R. (1981). Diagnosis and treatment of intracordal cysts. *Journal of Otolaryngology (Toronto), 10,* 363–370.

Moore, D. M., Berle, S., Hanson, D. G., & Ward, P. H. (1987). Videostroboscopy of the canine larynx. The effects of assymetrical laryngeal tension. *Laryngoscope, 97,* 543–553.

Morrison, M. D. (1984). A clinical voice laboratory, videotape and stroboscopic instrumentation. *Otolaryngology-Head and Neck Surgery, 92,* 487–488.

Musehold, A. (1898). Stroboskopische und photographische Studien über die Stellung der Stimmlippen im Brust und falsett-register. *Archivs für Laryngology und Rhinology, 7,* 1–21.

Oertel, M. J. (1895a). Das Laryngo-Stroboskop und die laryngostroboskopishe Untersuchung. *Archiv für Laryngology und Rhinology, 3,* 1–5.

Oertel, M. J. (1895b). Uumber eine neue laryngostroboscopische Untersuchungsmethode. *Münchener Medizinische Wochenschrift, 42,* 233–236.

Pakhmileviche, A. G. (1981). Elektronaia laringostroboskopicheskaia Kartina prinektrorykh. *Vestnik Oto-rino-laringologii (Moskva), 5,* 58–62.

Panconcelli, G. (1953). Das synchron-stroboskop nach Cremer. *HNO, 4,* 62.

Panconcelli-Calzia, G. (1929). Zeitlupenaufnahmen und Strobvokinematographie von Vorgangen im kehlkopf. *Zeitschrift für Laryngologie und Rhinologie, 17,* 394.

Pantiukhin, V. P. (1954). Novaia model 'stroboskopa. *Vestnik Oto-rino-laryngologii (Moskva), 16,* 5.

Pantiukhin, V. P. (1961). Stroboscopy in patients after laryngectomy. *Vestnik Oto-rino-laryngologii (Moskva), 23,* 69–73.

Pascher, W., Homoth, R., & Kruse, G. (1971). Verbesserung der visuellen Diagnostik in der Laryngologie und Phoniatrie. *HNO, 19,* 373–375.

Pasher, W., & Johannsen, H. S. (1975). Angewandte phoniatrie. I. Methodik der Stimmuntersuchung. *HNO, 23,* 84–90.

Pasher, W., & Neumann, G. (1976). Fiber-stroboskopie. Technik und Anwendungsmöglichkeiten. *Archives of Oto-Laryngology (Berlin), 213,* 464–465.

Perlman, H. B. (1945). Laryngeal strosobcopy. *Annals of Otology, Rhinology and Laryngology, 54,* 159–165.

Pedersen, M. F. (1977). Electroglottography compared with synchronized stroboscopy in the normal person. *Folia Phoniatrica, 29,* 191–199.

Peppard, R. C., & Bless, D. M. (1990). A method for improving measurement reliability in laryngeal videostroboscopy. *Journal of Voice, 4,* 280–285.

Peppard, R., Bless, D. M., & Milenkovic, P. (1988). Comparison of young adult singers and nonsingers with vocal nodules. *Journal of Voice, 2,* 250–260.

Pollak-Rudin, R., & Stein, L. (1932). Ein neues handliches Laryngostroboskop. *Wiener Medizinische Wochenschrift, 28,* 916–917.

Pomez, J., Fenelon, J., Chassaigne, M., & Dissez, A. (1969). L'examen phoniatrique chez quelques malades neurologiques. *Revue de Laryngologie, d'Otologie, et de Rhinologie, 90,* 375–383.

Powell, L. S. (1934). Laryngostrobscope. *Archives of Otolaryngology, 19,* 708–710.

Powell, L. S. (1935). The laryngo-stroboscope in clinical examination of the larynx. *Eye Ear Nose and Throat Monthly, 14,* 265.

Prytz, S. (1987). Layrngeal videostrobscopy. *Ear Nose Throat Journal (Suppl. Entechnology), 5.*

Prytz, S. (1989). Larygostroboscopy. Pamphlet. Naerum, Denmark: Brüel & Kjaer.

Raes, J., Lebrun, Y., & Clement, P. (1986). Videostroboscopy of the larynx. *Acta Oto-laryngologica (Stockholm), 40,* 421–425.

Raisova, V. (1988). Fiberoptische Laryngoskopie in der phoniatrischen Praxis. *Proceedings of the 15th UEP Congress,* Erlangen, Germany.

Rakhmilevich, A. G., & Lavrova, E. V. (1971). Phonopedic therapy and stroboscopy of patients with affection of the inferior laryngeal nerve. *Otorhinolaryngology, 33,* 10–12.

Rammage, L. A., Peppard, R. C., & Bless, D. M. (1992). Aerodynamic, laryngoscopic, and perceptual acoustic characteristics in dysphonic females with posterior glottal chinks: A retrospective study. *Journal of Voice, 6,* 64–78.

Rasinger, G. A., Frank, F., Neuwirth-Riedl, K., Wascher, K., & Gajsek, M. (1986). Erweiterte Einsatzgebieten von flexibilen und starren optiken in der laryngologie (p. 46). *Proceedings of the 13th Union of European Phoniatricians Congress,* Vienna, Austria.

Rohrs, M., Pascher, W., & Ocker, C. (1985). Untersuchungen über das Schwingungsverhalten der Stimmlippen in verschiedenen Registerbereichen mit unterschiedlichen stroboskopischen Techniken. *Folia Phoniatrica, 37,* 113–118.

Saito, S. (1973). Microchirurgie stroboscopique du larynx. *Revue d'Laryngologie, d'Otologie, et de Rhinologie (Bordeaux), 94,* 9–10.

Saito, S. (1977). Phonosurgery. Basic study on the mechanism of phonation and endolaryngeal microsurgery. *Otologia (Fukuoka), 23,* 171–184.

Saito, S., Fukuda, H., & Kitahara, S. (1975). Stroboscopic microsurgery of the larynx. *Archives of Otolaryngology, 101,* 196–201.

Saito, S., Fukuda, H., & Kitahara, S. (1976). Functional microsurgery of the larynx. *Journal of the Japan Bronchoesophagological Society, 27,* 8–16.

Saito, S., Fukuda, H., Kitahara, S., & Kokawa, N. (1978). Stroboscopic observation of vocal fold vibration with fiberoptics. *Folia Phoniatrica, 30,* 241–244.

Saito, S., Isogai, Y., & Fukuda, H. (1981). A newly developed laryngotelescope. *Journal of the Japan Bronchoesophagological Society, 32,* 328–331.

Salivon, L. G., & Kirina, N. I. (1972). Stroboscopy in malignant tumors of the larynx in the post-radiation period. *Zhurnal Ushnykh, Nosovykh i Govykh Boleznei, 32,* 74–76.

Sataloff, R. (1987a). Care of the professional voice. *Ear Nose Throat Journal, Special Issue, 66.*

Sataloff, R. T., Spiegel, J. R., Carroll, L. M., Schiebel, B. R., Darby, K. S., & Rulnick, R. K. (1987). Strobovideolaryngoscopy in professional voice users: Results and clinical value. *Journal of Voice, 1,* 359–364.

Sataloff, R. T., Spiegel, J. R., & Hawkshaw, M. J. (1991). Strobovideolaryngoscopy: Results and clinical value. *Annals of Otology, Rhinology, and Laryngology, 100,* 725–727.

Sawashima, M., Totsuka, G., Kobayashi, T., & Hirose, M. (1968). Reconstructive surgery for hoarseness due to unilateral vocal cord paralysis. *Archives of Otolaryngology, 87,* 289.

Schlossauer, B., & Timcke, R. (1956). Stroboscopic studies in hemilaryngectomized patients. *Archiv für Ohren-Nasen- und Kehlkopfheilkunde, 168,* 404–413.

Schonharl, E. (1952). Significance of laryngostroboscopy for practicing otorhinolaryngologists. *Laryngology Rhinology and Otology, 31,* 383–386.

Schonharl, E. (1954). Stroboscopic study in myxedema. *Archivs für Ohren- Nasen- und Kehlkopfheilkunde, 165,* 633–635.

Schonharl, E. (1956). New stroboscope with automatic regulation of frequency and recent results of its application to study of vocal cord vibrations in dysphonias of various origins. *Reviews of Laryngology, 77,* 476–481.

Schonharl, E. (1960a). *Die stroboskopie in der praktischen laryngologie.* Stuttgart: Georg Thieme Verlag.

Schonharl, E. (1960b). Zur stroboskopischen diagnostik von Stimmbandkarzinom und Tuberkulose. *Aktuelle Probleme der Phoniatrie und Logapaedie, 1,* 118–124.

Schuerenberg, B. (1988). Vibratory patterns of the vocal folds under pathological conditions. *Proceedings of the 15th Union of European Phoniatricians Congress* (pp. 201–205) [Erlangen]. Köln: Deutsche Artze Verlag.

Schuerenberg, B., & Moser, M. (1986). Entwicklung und derzeitiger Stand der TV-farbstroboskopie. *Proceedings of the 13th UEP Congress* (p. 24), Vienna.

Schultz-Coulon, H. J., & Klingholz, F. (1988). Objektive und semiobjektive Untersuchungsmethoden der Stimme. *Proceedings of the 15th UEP Congress,* Erlangen, Germany.

Sedlackova, E. (1981). Stroboscopic data in relation to the development of voice in children. *Folia Phoniatrica, 33,* 81–92.

Seeman, M. (1921). Laryngostroboskopische Untersuchungen bei einseitiger Recurrensparese. *Monatsschrift für Ohrenheilkunde und Laryngo-Rhinologie, 55,* 1621–1634.

Segre, R. (1933). Vocal nodules as revealed by stroboscope. *Valsalva, 9,* 380–389.

Segre, R. (1970). *Fono Audiologica, 16,* 23.

Segre, R., & Salvatori, J. M. (1969). *Fono Audiologica, 15,* 191.

Seidner, W., Wendler, J., & Halbedl, G. (1972). Mikrostroboskopie. *Folia Phoniatrica, 24,* 81–85.

Sercarz, J. A., Berke, G. S., Arnstein, D., Gerratt, B., & Navidad, M. (1991). A new technique for quantiative measurement of laryngeal videostroboscopic images. *Archives of Otolaryngology-Head and Neck Surgery, 117,* 871–875.

Sercarz, J. A., Berke, J. S., Gerratt, B. R., Kreiman, J., Ming, Y., & Navidad, M. (1992). Synchronizing videostroboscopic images of human laryngeal vibration with physiological signals. *American Journal of Otolaryngology, 13,* 40–44.

Sercarz, J. A., Berke, G. S., Ming, Y., Gerratt, B. R., & Navidad, M. (1992). Videostroboscopy of human vocal fold paralysis. *Annals of Otology, Rhinology, and Laryngology, 101,* 567–577.

Shaikh, A., & Bless, D. M. Preliminary comparison of vocal fold vibration with strobotelescopic and strobofibroscopic examinations. *Proceedings of the International Conference on Voice, 2,* 9–14.

Siegert, C. (1972). Bemerkungen zum stroboskopischen Bild bei Kindern. *HNO, 20,* 181–184.

Simko, S., & Szabo, L. (1988). Die bedeutung der Stroboskopie für die Indikation microchirurgischer Eingriffe an den Stimmbandern. *Proceedings of the 15th Union of European Phoniatricians Congress [Erlangen].* Köln: Deutsche Artze Verlag.

Stern, H. (1935). Study of larynx and of voice by means of stroboscopic moving picture. *Monatsschrift für Ohrenheilkunde und Laryngo-Rhinologie, 69,* 648–652.

Stone, R. E., Jr., & Lingeman, R. E. (1987). A proposal for insurance coverage of laryngeal videoendoscopic and videostroboscopic examination. Unpublished manuscript. Indianapolis: Indiana University School of Medicine, Department of Otolaryngology-Head Neck Surgery.

Suzuki, Y., Saito, S., Hayasaki, H., & Murakami, Y. (1964). Comptes Rendus des Seances; Congres Française. *Société Française d'Oto-Rhino-Laryngologie et de Pathologie Cervico-Faciale, 67,* 752.

Svanholm, H., & Lindholm, H. (1988). Videodocumentation at laryngoscopy. *Acta Oto-laryngologica (Stockholm), 449,* 35.

Szentesi, D. I. (1972). Stroboscopic electron mirror microscopy at frequencies up to 100 MHz. *Journal of Physics E. Scientific Instruments, 5,* 563–567.

Tanabe, M., Kitajima, K., Gould, W. J., & Lambiase, A. (1975). Analysis of high-speed motion pictures of the vocal folds. *Folia Phoniatrica, 27,* 77–87.

Tarneaud, J. L. (1932). Les dyskinésies de la parole et du chant. *Annales d'Otolaryngologie et de Chirurgie Cervico-Faciale,* 864–890.

Tarneaud, J. L. (1933). Study of larynx and of voice by stroboscopy. *Clinique, 28,* 337–341.

Tarneaud, J. L. (1937). *La stroboscopie du larynx: Séméiologie stroboscopique des maladies du larynx et de la voix* (1 ère éd., p. 91). Paris: Médicales et N. Maloine.

Tarneaud, J. L. (1961). *Traité pratique de phonologie et de phoniatrie* (éme éd., p. 521). Paris: Maloine.

Tassini, G. (1966). Methods and possibilities of opaque laryngography. *Clinica Otorinolaryngoiatrica, 18,* 443–450.

Timcke, R. (1956a). Die Synchron-stroboskopie von menschlichen Stimmlippen bzw. Ähnlichen Schallquellen und Messung der Öffnungszeit. *Zeitschrift für Laryngologie und Rhinologie, 35,* 331–335.

Timcke, R. (1956b). Laryngostroboskopie Mittels eines neuartigen Synchronstroboskops. *Zeitschrift für Hals-, Nasen- und Kehlkopfheilkunde, 169,* 539–543.

Tischner, H. (1955). Vocal cord stroboscopy with automatic adjustment of frequency. *Archiv für Ohren-, Nasen- und Kehlkopfheilkunde, 167,* 524–529.

Trapp, T. K., & Berke, G. S. (1988). Photoelectric measurement of laryngeal paralyses correlated with videostroboscopy. *Laryngoscope, 98,* 486–492.

Van Clooster, R. (1973). Laryngomicrostroboscopy. *Minerva Otorinolaryngologica, 23,* 254–255.

van den Berg, J. W. (1954). Über die Koppelung bei Stimmbildung 1954. *Zeitschrift Phonetik, 8,* 281–293.

van den Berg, J. W., & Tan, T. S. (1959). Données nouvelles sur la fonction laryngée. *Journal Françiase d'Oto-Rhino-Laryngologie, Audiophonologie, et Chirurgie Maxillo-Faciale, 8,* 103–111.

Vallancien, B. (1954). Le strobophone. *Transactions de la Societé de Laryngologie des Hôpitaux de Paris.*

Vasilenko, Y. S. (1972). Significance of individual indices of vibratory cycle of the vocal folds in general assessment of the stroboscopic picture. *Vestnik Oto-rino-laryngologii (Moskva), 34,* 63–68.

Vasilenko, Y. S., & Ivanchenko, G. F. (1978). Microlaryngostrobic examination of patients with functional diseases of the larynx. *Vestnik Oto-rino-laryngologii (Moskva), 39,* 69–73.

Verhulst, J. L. (1984a). L'examen dynamique des cordes vocales: Comparison entre la laryngoscopie avec l'endoscope rigide et la fibroscopie. *Revue de Laryngologie Otologie Rhinologie (Bordeaux), 105,* 437–439.

Verhulst, J. L. (1984b). La vidéo laryngostroboscopie. *Bordeaux Medical, 17,* 1037–1039.

von Leden, H. V. (1961). The electric synchron-stroboscope: Its value for the practicing laryngologist. *Annals of Otology, Rhinology, and Laryngology, 70,* 881–893.

von Leden, H. V., Moore, P., & Timcke, R. (1960). Laryngeal vibrations: III. The pathologic larynx. *Archives of Otology, 71,* 1232–1250.

Voronina, E. M., & Shtumer, Y. F. (1939). Strobofaradizator. *Zhurnal Ushnykh Nosovykh, i Gorlovikh Boleznei*, 16, 258–263.

Wangler, M. A., & Weaver, J. M. (1984). A method to facilitate fiberoptic laryngoscopy. [Letter to the editor]. *Anesthesiology*, 61, 111.

Ward, P. H., & Berci, G. (1982). Observations on the pathogenesis of chronic non-specific pharyngitis and laryngitis. *Laryngoscope*, 92, 1377–1382.

Ward, P. H., Berci, G., & Galcaterra, T. C. (1982). Advances in endoscopic examination of the respiratory system. *Annals of Otology, Rhinology, and Laryngology*, 91, 354–358.

Ward, P. H., Hanson, D. G., Gerratt, B. R., & Berke, G. S. (1989). Current and future horizons in laryngeal and voice research. *Annals of Otology, Rhinology, and Laryngology*, 98, 145–152.

Watanabe, H., Shin, T., & Matsuo, K. (1986). A new computer-analyzing system for clinical use with the strobovideoscope. *Archives of Otolaryngology*, 112, 978–981.

Weiss, D. (1932). Die Laryngostroboskopie. *Zeitschrift für Laryngologie, Rhinologie, Otologie und ihre Grenzgebiete*, 22, 391–418.

Wendler, J. (1967). Die Bedeutung der Stimmstärke bei der Stroboskopischen Untersuchung. *Folia Phoniatrica*, 19(2), 73–88.

Wendler, J. (1976). *Practical hints for the application of laryngostroboscopy*. Dresden: VEB Turk.

Wendler, J. (1988). Consideraciones sobre una instrumentacion razonnable para el diagnostico de voz en la practica clinica. *Revue Logopaedia Foniatrica et Audiologica*, 8, 49–53.

Wendler, J. (1992). Stroboscopy [Special Article]. *Journal of Voice*, 6, 149–154.

Wendler, J., Koppen, K., & Fischer, S. (1987). The validity of stroboscopic data in terms of quantitative measures. *Acta Phoniatrica Latina*, 11, 7–12.

Wendler, J., Koppen, K., Fischer, S., & Cebulla, M. (1988). On the clinical relevance of vibratory parameters in laryngostroboscopy. *Proceedings of the 15th Union of European Phoniatricians Congress* [Erlangen]. Köln: Deutscher Artze Verlag.

Wendler, J., Otto, C., & Nawka, T. H. (1983). Stroboglottometrie — Eine neues Verfahren zur Schwingungsanalyse der Stimmlippen. *HNO-Praxis*, 8, 263–268.

Wendler, J., & Seidler, W. (1988). Methoden und ergebnisse der Phonochirurgie. *Zeitschrift für Klinische Medizin*, 46, 101–103.

West, R. (1935). A view of the larynx through a new stroboscope. *Quarterly Journal of Speech*, 21, 355.

White, J. F., & Knight, R. E. (1984). Office videofiberoptic laryngoscopy. *Laryngoscope*, 94, 1166–1169.

Winckel, F. (1954a). Neuentwicklung eines Lichtblitz-Stroboskops für die Laryngologie. *HNO*, 4, 210.

Winckel, F. (1954b). Improved stroboscopic technique for examination. *Archiv Ohren-, Nasen- und Kehlkopfheilkunde*, 165, 585–586.

Witzig, E., Cornut, G., Bouchayer, M., Roch, J. B., & Loire, R. (1983). Ètude anatomoclinique et traitement des kystes epidermoides et des sulcus de la corde vocale (à propos de 157 cas). *Les Cahiers d'Oto Rhino Laryngologie*, 18, 766–780.

Witzig, E., Cornut, G., Bouchayer, M., Roch, J. B., & Loire, R. (1985). Le kyste muqueux par retention de la corde vocale. Serie anatomoclinique de 32 cas. *Rundschau Medicine (PRAXIS) (Schweiz)*, 21, 554–557.

Wolfe, R. (1987). *Stroboscopy*. Unpublished manuscript.

Yana, D. (1969). La stroboscopie du larynx: À propos d'un nouveaux stroboscope, le stroborama type. *Annals of Otolaryngologie Chirurgie Cervicofaciale*, 86, 589–592.

Yanagisawa, E. (1983). Videolaryngoscopy: A comparison of fiberscopic and telescopic documentation. *Annals of Otology, Rhinology, and Laryngology*, 92, 430–436.

Yanagisawa, E., Godley, F., & Muta, H. (1987). Selection of video cameras for stroboscopic videolaryngoscopy. *Annals of Otology, Rhinology, and Laryngology*, 96, 578–585.

Yanagisawa, E., Owens, T. W., Strothers, G., & Honda, K. (1983). Videolaryngoscopy: A comparison of fiberscopic and telescopic documentation. *Otology, Rhinology, and Laryngology*, 92, 430–436.

Yoshida, Y. (1977). An improved model of laryngo-stroboscope. *Otolaryngology*, 49, 663–669.

Yoshida, Y. (1979). A video-tape recording system for laryngostroboscopy. *Journal of the Japan Bronchoesophagological Society*, 30, 1–5.

Yoshida, Y., Hirano, M., & Nakajima, T. (1979). An improved model of laryngo-stroboscope. *Journal of the Japan Bronchoesophagological Society*, 30, 6–12.

Yoshida, Y., Hirano, M., Yoshida, T., & Tateishi, O. (1985). Strobofiberscopic colour video recording of vocal fold vibrations. *Journal of Laryngology and Otology*, 99, 795–800.

SEDATION AND TOPICAL ANESTHETICS

American Speech-Language-Hearing Association Ad Hoc Committee on Advances in Clinical Practice. (1992). Sedation and topical anesthetics in audiology and speech-language pathology. *ASHA*, 34, 41–42.

Catalano, G., Rossi, M. M. Y., & Disceglie, P. (1963). *Clinical Otorhinolaryngiatrica*, 15, 197.

Colman, M. F., & Reynolds, R. (1985). The use of topical

cocaine to prevent laryngospasm after general anesthesia on endoscopy procedures. *Laryngoscope, 95,* 474.

Kiowa, S. (1973). Anesthesia for new functional laryngeal microsurgery with droperidol and fentanyl. *Matsui. Japanese Journal of Anesthesiology, 22,* 545–552.

Raj, P. P., Forestner, J., Watson, T. D., Morris, R. E., & Jenkins, M. T. (1974). Technics for fiberoptic laryngoscopy in anaesthesia. *Anaesthesia and Analgesia, 53,* 708–714.

ANATOMY AND PHYSIOLOGY ISSUES RELATED TO STROBOSCOPIC RECORDING INTERPRETATIONS

Colton, R. H., Casper, J. K., Brewer, D. W., & Conture, E. G. (1989). Digital processing of laryngeal images: A preliminary report. *Journal of Voice, 3,* 132–142.

Grant, J. C. B. (1958). *A method of anatomy* (p. 783). Baltimore: Williams & Wilkins.

Hirano, M. (1974). Morphological structure of the vocal cord as a vibrator and its variations. *Folia Phoniatrica, 26,* 89–94.

Hirano, M. (1981b). Structure of the vocal fold in normal and diseased states: Anatomical and physical study. In *Proceedings of the Conference on the Assessment of Vocal Pathology, American Speech-Language-Hearing Association Report, 11,* 69.

Hirano, M., Kakita, Y., Kawasaki, H., & Matsushita, H. (1977). *Vocal fold vibration: Behavior of the layer-structured vibrator in normal and pathological conditions.* (16 mm film also available on videotape). New York: The Voice Foundation.

Hirano, M., Kakita, Y., Ohmaru, K., & Kurita, S. (1982). Structure and mechanical properties of the vocal fold. In N. J. Lass (Ed.), *Speech and language: Advances in basic research and practice* (pp. 271–297). New York: Academic Press.

Hirano, M., Kurita, S., Matsuo, K., & Nagata, K. (1981). Vocal fold polyp and polypoid vocal fold (Reinke's edema). *Journal of Research in Singing, 4,* 33–44.

Hirano, M., Matsushita, H., Kawasaki, H., Yoshida, Y., & Koike, Y. (1974). Vibrations of the vocal cords with unilateral polyp. An ultra high speed cinematographic study. *Journal of Otolaryngology of Japan, 77,* 593–610.

Hirano, M., & Stevens, K. (Eds.). (1981). Vocal fold physiology. *Vocal Fold Physiology Conference Proceedings.* Tokyo: University of Tokyo Press.

Hiroto, I. (1966). The mechanism of phonation, its pathophysiologic aspects. *Oto Rhino Laryngology Clinic, Kyoto, 59,* 229–291.

METHODS

American Speech-Language-Hearing Association Ad Hoc Committee on Advances in Clinical Practice. (1992a). Sedation and topical anesthetics in audiology and speech-language pathology. *ASHA, 34,* 41–42.

American Speech-Language-Hearing Association. (1992b). Vocal tract visualization and imaging. *ASHA, 34,* 37–40.

Andrews, J. H., Jr., & Gould, W. J. (1977). Laryngeal and nasopharyngeal indirect telescope. *Annals of Otology, Rhinology, and Laryngology, 86,* 627.

Baken, J. R. (1987). *Clinical measurement of speech and voice.* Boston: College-Hill Press.

Bartell, T., Bless, D. M., & Ford, C. N. (1986). Rating forms for videostroboscopic analysis of voice production. *Proceedings of the International Association of Logopedics and Phoniatrics Conference on Voice, 2,* 15–21.

Bastian, R. W. (1987a). Laryngeal image feedback for voice disorder patients. *Journal of Voice, 1,* 279–282.

Bastian, R. W. (1987b). Laryngeal videostroboscopy and photography for the diagnosis and management of voice disorders. *Insights in Otolaryngology, 2.*

Blair, R. L., Berry, H., & Briant, T. D. R. (1978). Laryngeal electromyography: Techniques and application. *Otolaryngologic Clinics of North America, 2,* 325–346.

Bless, D. M., & Baken, R. J. (1992). Assessment of voice. *Journal of Voice, 6,* 95–97.

Bridgeman, B., & Klassen, H. (1983). On the origin of stroboscopic induced motion. *Perception and Psychoacoustics, 34,* 149–154.

Brodie, K., Colton, R. H., & Swisher, L. (1988). *Reliability of inverse filtered and EGG measurements of vocal function.* Unpublished manuscript.

Colton, R. H., Brewer, D. W., & Rothenberg, M. (1983). Evaluating vocal fold function. *Journal of Otolaryngology, 12,* 291–294.

Colton, R. H., & Casper, J. K. (1990). *Understanding voice problems: A physiological perspective for diagnosis and treatment.* Baltimore: Williams & Wilkins.

Colton, R. H., Casper, J. K., Brewer, D. W., & Conture, E. G. (1989). Digital processing of laryngeal images: A preliminary report. *Journal of Voice, 3,* 132–142.

Luchsinger, R., & Nielson, E. (1991). Measurement of the length of the vocal cords during an increase in pitch of a note. *Folia Phoniatrica, 13,* 1–12.

Morrison, M. D., Nichol, H., & Rammage, L. A. (1986).

Diagnostic criteria in functional dysphonia. *Laryngoscope, 94,* 1.

Tassini, G., & Pazzaglia, P. G. (1966). *Valsalva, 42,* 67.

ENDOSCOPY

American Speech-Language-Hearing Association. (1992b). Vocal tract visualization and imaging. *ASHA, 34,* 37–40.

Andrews, Jr., A. H., & Gould, W. J. (1977). Laryngeal and nasopharyngeal indirect telescope. *Annals of Otology, Rhinology, and Laryngology, 86,* 627.

Asahi Optical Company, Ltd. *Pentax Curved Laryngotelescope.* Tokyo, Japan.

Brewer, D. W., & McCall, G. (1974). Visible laryngeal changes during voice therapy: Fiberoptic study. *Annals of Otology Rhinology, and Laryngology, 83,* 423–427.

Cantarella, G. (1987). Value of flexible videolaryngoscopy in the study of laryngeal morphology and functions. *Journal of Voice, 1,* 353–358.

Casper, J. K., Brewer, D. W., & Colton, R. H. (1987a). Pitfalls and problems in flexible fiberoptic videolaryngoscopy. *Journal of Voice, 1,* 347–352.

Casper, J. K., Brewer, D. W., & Colton, R. H. (1987b). Variations in normal human laryngeal anatomy and physiology as viewed fiberscopically. *Journal of Voice, 1,* 180–185.

Centers for Disease Control Morbidity and Mortality Weekly Report. (1988, June). *Perspectives in Disease Prevention and Health Promotion, 37,* 377–388.

Dancygier, H., Wurbs, D., & Classen, M. (1981). A new method for the endoscopic determination of gastrointestinal ulcer area. *Endoscopy, 13,* 214–216.

Davidson, T. M., Bone, R. C., & Nahum, A. M. (1974). Flexible fiberoptic laryngobronchoscopy. *Laryngoscope, 84,* 1876–1882.

Dellon, A. L., Clifford, A. H., and Chretien, D. B. (1975). Fiberoptic endoscopy in the head and neck region. *Plastic and Reconstructive Surgery, 55,* 466–471.

Gould, W. J. (1973). The Gould laryngoscope. *Journal of the American Academy of Ophthalmology and Otolaryngology, 77,* 38–141.

Gould, W. J., Kojima, H., & Lambaise, A. (1979). A technique for stroboscopic examination of the vocal folds using fiberoptics. *Archives of Otolaryngology, 105,* 285.

Hirano, M. (1988). *Endolaryngeal microsurgery.* In G. M. English (Ed.), *Otolaryngology* (Vol. 3, pp. 1–22). Philadelphia: J. B. Lippincott.

Izdebski, K., Ross, J. C., & Klein, J. C. (1990). Transoral rigid laryngovideostroboscopy (phonoscopy). *Seminars in Speech and Language, 1,* 16–26.

Katzenberg, B. (1983). Endoscopic photography in otolaryngology. *Journal of Biological Photography, 49,* 101–107.

Lindestad, P. A., & Sodersten, M. (1968). Laryngeal and pharyngeal behavior in countertenor and baritone singing — A videofiberscopic study. *Journal of Voice, 2,* 132–139.

McFarlane, S. C., & Watterson, T. L. (1990). Vocal nodules: Endoscopic study of their variations and treatment. *Seminars in Speech and Language, 1,* 47–59.

Painter, C., & Komiyama, S. (1987). On buying a telescope for videolaryngoscopy. *Laryngoscope, 97,* 758.

Pascher, W., & Neumann, P. (1976). Fiber-stroboskopie. Technik und Anwendungsmöglichkeiten. *Archives of Oto-Laryngology (Berlin), 213,* 464–465.

Paschow, M. S., & Mattucci, K. F. (1983). Direct laryngoscopy: A retrospective analysis. *International Surgery, 68,* 331–335.

Perlman, H. B. (1945). Laryngeal stroboscopy. *Annals of Otology, Rhinology, and Laryngology, 54,* 159–165.

Raisova, V. (1988). Fiberoptische Laryngoskopie in der phoniatrischen Praxis. *Proceedings of the 15th UEP Conference* [Erlangen]. Köln: Deutscher Artze Verlag.

Saito, S., Fukuda, H., Kitihara, S., & Isogai, Y. (1984). Curved laryngotelescope. *Laryngoscope, 94,* 1103–1105.

Sawashima, M., Abramson, A. S., Cooper, F. S., & Lisker, L. (1970). Observing laryngeal adjustment during running speech by use of a fiberoptics system. *Phonetica, 22,* 193–201.

Sawashima, M., & Hirose, H. (1968). New laryngoscope technique by use of fiber-optics. *Journal of the Acoustical Society of America, 43,* 168–169.

Schafermeyer, R. W. (1983). Fiberoptic laryngoscopy in the emergency department. *American Journal of Emergency Medicine, 2,* 160–163.

Selkin, S. G. (1983a). Flexible fiberoptics for laryngeal photography. *Laryngoscope, 93,* 657–658.

Selkin, S. G. (1983b). The otolaryngologist and flexible fiberoptics: Photographic consideration. *Journal of Otolaryngology, 12,* 223–227.

Selkin, S. G. (1984). Other clinical applications of flexible fiberoptic endoscopy. *Cleft Palate Journal, 21,* 29–32.

Shaikh, A., & Bless, D. M. (1986). Preliminary comparison of vocal fold vibration with strobotelescopic and strobofibroscopic examinations. *Proceedings of the International Conference on Voice, 2,* 9–14.

Silberman, H. D., Wilf, H., & Tucker, J. A. (1967). Flexible fiberoptic nasopharyngolaryngoscope. *Annals of Oto-Rhino-Laryngology, 85,* 640–645.

Stern, H. (1935). Study of the larynx and of voice by means of videostroboscopic moving picture. *Mon-*

atsschrift für Ohrenheilkunde und Laryngo-Rhinologie, 69, 648–652.

Svanholm, H., & Lindholm, H. (1988). Videodocumentation at laryngoscopy. *Acta Oto-laryngologica (Stockholm),* 449, 35.

Tobin, H. A. (1990). Office fiberoptic laryngeal photography. *Otolaryngology-Head Neck Surgery,* 88, 172–173.

Wangler, M. A., & Weaver, J. M. (1984). A method to facilitate fiberoptic laryngoscopy. [Letter to the editor]. *Anesthesiology,* 61, 111.

Watterson, T. L., & McFarlane, S. C. (1990). Transnasal videoendoscopy of the velopharyngeal port mechanism. *Seminars in Speech and Language,* 11, 27–37.

Watterson, T. L., McFarlane, S. C., & Brophy, J. W. (1990a). Some issues and ethics in oral and nasal videoendoscopy. *Seminars in Speech and Language,* 11, 1–7.

Watterson, T. L., McFarlane, S. C., & Brophy, J. W. (1990b). Transnasal videoendoscopy of the laryngeal mechanism. *Seminars in Speech and Language,* 11, 8–15.

Weir, N., & Bassett, L. (1987). Out patient fibreoptic nasolaryngoscopy and videostroboscopy. *Journal of the Royal Society of Medicine (London),* 80, 229–230.

Welch, A. R. (1982). The practical and economic value of flexible system laryngoscopy. *Journal of Laryngology and Otology,* 96, 1125–1129.

White, J. F., & Knight, R. E. (1984). Office videofiberoptic laryngoscopy. *Laryngoscope,* 94, 1166–1169.

Williams, G. T., Farquharson, I. M., & Anthony, J. K. (1975). Fiberoptic laryngoscopy in the assessment of laryngeal disorders. *Journal of Laryngology and Otology,* 89, 299–316.

Wilson, F. B., Kudryk, W. H., & Sych, J. A. (1986). The development of flexible fiberoptic video nasoendoscopy (FFVN): Clinical, teaching, research applications. *ASHA,* 28, 25–30.

Witton, T. H. (1981). An introduction to the fiberoptic laryngoscope. *Canadian Anesthetists Society Journal,* 28, 475–478.

Yanagisawa, E. (1981). Office telescopic photography of the larynx. *Annals of Otology, Rhinology, and Laryngology,* 91, 354–358.

Yanagisawa, E., Casuccio, J. R., & Suzuki, M. (1981). Videolaryngoscopy using a rigid telescope and video home system color camera. *Annals of Otology, Rhinology, and Laryngology,* 90, 346–350.

Yanagisawa, E., Owens, T. W., Strothers, G., & Honda, K. (1983). Videolaryngoscopy: A comparison of fiberscopic and telescopic documentation. Annals of Otology, Rhinology, and Laryngology, 92, 430–436.

Zwitman, D. H. (1990). Utilization of transoral endoscopy to assess velopharyngeal closure. *Seminars in Speech and Language,* 11, 38–46.

BACKGROUND AND PRINCIPLES

Bernthal, J. E., & Beukelman, D. R. (1978). Intraoral air pressure during the production of /p/ and /b/ by children, youths, and adults. *Journal of Speech and Hearing Research,* 21, 361–371.

Blitzer, A., Lovelace, R. E., Brin, M. F., Fahn, S., & Fink, M. E. (1985). Electromyographic findings in vocal laryngeal dystonia (spastic dysphonia). *Annals of Otology, Rhinology and Laryngology,* 94, 591-594.

Bouchayer, M., Cornut, G., Witzig, E., Loire, R., Roch, J. B., & Bastian, R. (1985). Epidermoid cysts, sulci and mucosi bridges of the true vocal cord: A report of 157 cases. *Laryngoscope,* 95, 1087–1094.

Brewer, D. W. (1989). Voice research: The next ten years. *Journal of Voice,* 3, 7–17.

Broda-Masiuk, D. (1984, November). *Flexible fiberoptic video nasendoscopy: A tool in voice disorder management.* Paper presented at the American Speech-Language-Hearing Association Annual Convention, San Francisco, CA.

Brüel & Kjaer Co. (1984) *Rino-larynx Stroboscope, Type 4914.* Marlborough, MA: Brüel & Kjaer.

Coleman, R. F., Mabis, J. H., & Hinson, J. K. (1977). Fundamental frequency-sound pressure level profiles of adult male and female voices. *Journal of Speech and Hearing Research,* 20, 197–204.

Edgerton, H. E. (1970). *Electronic flash, strobe.* New York: McGraw-Hill.

Ertl, E., & Stein, L. (1936). History of motorless laryngostroboscopy. *Monatsschrift für Ohrenheilkunde und Laryngo-Rhinologie,* 70, 1463–1464.

Evers, W., Racz, G. B., Glazer, J., & Dobkin, A. B. (1967). Orahesive as a protection for the teeth during general anaesthesia and endoscopy. *Canadian Anaesthetists Society Journal,* 14, 123–128.

Farnsworth, D. W. (1940). *High speed motion pictures of human vocal cords.* Bell Telephone Laboratories.

Farr, J., & Silveria, R. (1961). *Transactions of the Pacific Coast Otological Society,* 309.

Faure, M. A., & Muller, A. (1992). Stroboscopy [Special Article]. *Journal of Voice,* 6, 139–148.

Ferrein, A. (1741). De la formation de la voix de l' homme. *Histoire de la Société Royale de Médicine (Paris),* 409–432.

Finlay, D. (1982). Stroboscopic motion in depth. *Perception,* 11, 733–741.

Frank, F. (1986). Optics in phoniatrics. *Proceedings of the XIII Congress Union of European Phoniatricians Congress,* Vienna, Austria

Fritzell, B., & Fant, G. (1986). Voice acoustics and dysphonia. *Journal of Phonetics,* 14, 351–359.

Fujita, H., & Fujita, T. (1981). *Textbook of histology, Part 1.* Tokyo: Igaku Shoin Ltd.

Garcia, M. (1855). Observations of the human voice. *Philosophical Magazine Journal of Science 10,* 511–513.

Gerratt, B. R., Hanson, D. G., & Berke, G. S. (1988). Laryngeal configuration associated with glottography. *American Journal of Otolaryngology, 9,* 173–179.

Hala, B., & Honnty, L. (1931). Cinematography of vocal cords by means of stroboscope and great speed. *Otolaryngologia Slavica, 3,* 1–12.

Halbedl, G. (1964). Grundlagen der technik der Kehlfopfstroboskopie. In *Handbuch Medizin Elektronik, Teil II.* Berlin: VEB Technik.

Hartmann, H. G. (1985). *Diagnosis using stroboscopy.* Naerum, Denmark: Brüel et Kjaer.

Hirano, M., Matsushita, H., Kawasaki, H., Yoshida, Y., & Koike, Y. (1974). Vibration of the vocal cords with unilateral polyp. An ultra high speed cinematographic study. *Journal of Otolaryngology of Japan, 77,* 593–610.

Hirano, M., Yoshida, Y., Matsushita, H., & Nakajima, T. (1974). An apparatus for high speed cinematography of the vocal folds. *Annals of Otology, Rhinology, and Laryngology, 83,* 12–18.

Hirose, H. (1988). High-speed digital imaging of vocal fold vibration. *Acta Oto-laryngologica (Stockholm), 458,* 151–153.

Hollien, H. (1964). In *Proceedings of the 5th International Congress of Science* (Munich), 362.

Ishizaka, K., & Isshiki, N. (1976). Computer simulation of pathological vocal cord vibration. *Journal of the Acoustical Society of America, 60,* 1193–1198.

Jephcott, A. (1984). The Macintosh Laryngoscope. A historical note on its clinical and commercial development. *Anaesthesia, 39,* 474–479.

Kallen, L. A. (1932). Laryngostroboscopy in the practice of otolaryngology. *Archives of Otolaryngology, 16,* 791–807.

Kallen, L. A., & Polin, H. S. (1934). A physiological stroboscope. *Science, 80,* 592.

Kallen, L. A., & Polin, H. S. (1937). Ein physiologisches stroboskop. *Monatsschrift für Ohrenheilkunde und Laryngo-Rhinologie, 71,* 1177–1181.

Karnell, M. P. (1989). Synchronized videostroboscopy and electroglottography. *Journal of Voice, 3,* 68–75.

Kivenson, G. (1965). *Industrial stroboscopy.* New York: Hayden Book Company, Inc.

Koike, Y. (1973). Application of some acoustic measures for the evaluation of laryngeal dysfunction. *Studia Phonologica, 7,* 17–23.

Koike, Y. (1975). High-speed photography of the larynx and film data processing. *Canadian Journal of Otolaryngology, 4,* 800–805.

Koike, Y. (1979). Diagnosis of voice disorders. *Nippon Jibiinkoka Gakkai Kaiho, 82,* 1434–1437.

Kotby, M. N., Barakah, M. S., El-Ella, M. Y., Khidr, A. A., & Hegazi, M. A. (1989). Aerodynamic analysis of voice disorders. In *Proceedings of the XIV World Congress of Otorhinolaryngology Head and Neck Surgery,* Madrid, Spain.

Krahulec, I. (1970). Importance of stroboscopy in laryngology. *Ceskoslovenska Otolaryngologica, 19,* 29–31.

Lafon, J. C. (1959). *L'impulsion acoustique unité de phonation et d'audition* (p. 248). LVIE Congres Français d'Oto-Rhino-Laryngologie. Paris: Arnette.

Landeau, M. (1953). *La voix.* Paris: Maloine.

Laver, J. (1976). Perceptual dimensions and acoustical correlates of pathological voices. *Acta Otolaryngologica (Suppl. 338).*

Leeper, H. A., & Wilkins, C. (1985). *VOT in 75-year-old females.* Paper presented at the Canadian Speech and Hearing Association Meeting.

Luchsinger, R., & Turetschek, G. (1950). *Folia Phoniatrica, 2, 5.*

MacKay, D. M. (1970). Fragmentation of binocular fusion in stroboscopic illumination. *Nature, 227,* 518.

Marcos, J., & Pedrosa, C. (1969). Revista medica del hospital general. *Asturias, 4,* 14.

Matsushita, H. (1975). The vibratory mode of the vocal folds in the excised larynx. *Folia Phoniatrica, 27,* 7–18.

Mihashi, K. (1977). Investigations of phonatory function following vertical partial laryngectomy. *Otologia Fukuoka, 23,* 786–806.

Milner, M., Brennan, P. K., & Wilberforce, C. B. (1973). Stroboscopic polaroid photography in clinical studies of human locomotion. *South African Medical Journal, 47,* 948–950.

Minnigerode, B. (1967). The defiguration phenomenon in motion perception and its effect on stroboscopic laryngoscopy. *Laryngologie Rhinologie und Otologie, 101,* 33–38.

Minnigerode, B. (1969). Die Invertierbarkeit dreidimensionaler Körper und ihre Bedeutung für die objektive Laryngoscopie. *Monatsschrift für Ohrenheilkunde und Laryngo-Rhinologie, 103,* 210–217.

Morrison, M. D. (1984). A clinical voice laboratory, videotape and stroboscopic instrumentaion. *Otolaryngology-Head and Neck Surgery, 92,* 487–488.

Motta, G., Cesari, U., Iengo, M., & Motta, G., Jr. (1990). Clinical application of electroglottography. *Folia Phoniatrica, 42,* 111–117.

Muller, J. (1840). *Handbuch der Physiologie des Menschen. Vol. 2. von der Stimme und Sprache* (pp. 133–248).

Netsell, R., Shaughnessey, A. L., & Lotz, W. K. (1983). Laryngeal aerodynamics for selected vocal pathologies.

Abstracts of the Association of Research Otolaryngology, 80.

Noscoe, N. J., Bourcin, A. M., Brown, N. J., & Berry, R. J. (1983). Examination of vocal fold movement by ultrashort pulse X radiography. *British Journal of Radiology, 56,* 641–645.

Ocker, C., Pascher, W., & Rohrs, M. (1983). Investigations of the vibration modes of the vocal cords during different registers. *Proceedings of the Stockholm Music Acoustics Conference, 1,* 239–246.

Oertel, M. J. (1895a). Das Laryngo-Stroboskop und die laryngostroboskopische Untersuchung. *Archivs für Laryngology und Rhinology, 3,* 1–5.

Olesen, H. P. (1986). *The rhino-larynx stroboscope type 4914 used with other instruments* (p. 12). Stockholm: Brüel & Kjaer.

Padovan, I. F., Christman, M. T., Hamilton, L. H., & Darling, R. J. (1973). Indirect microlaryngostroboscopy. *Laryngoscope, 83,* 2035–2041.

Pederson, M. F. (1977). Electroglottography compared with synchronized stroboscopy in the normal person. *Folia Phoniatrica, 29,* 191–199.

Pershall, K. E., & Boone, D. R. (1987). Supraglottic contribution to voice quality. *Journal of Voice, 1,* 186–190.

Powell, L. S. (1934). Laryngostroboscope. *Archives of Otolaryngology, 19,* 708–710.

Powell, L. S. (1935). The laryngostroboscope in clinical examination of the larynx. *Eye Ear Nose and Throat Monthly, 14,* 265.

Prytz, S. (1987). Laryngeal videostroboscopy. *Ear Nose Throat Journal (Suppl. Entechnology),* 5.

Prytz, S. (1989). *Laryngostroboscopy.* Pamphlet. Naerum, Denmark: Brüel & Kjaer.

Raes, J., Lebrun, Y., & Clement, P. (1986). Videostroboscopy of the larynx. *Acta Oto-laryngologica (Stockholm), 40,* 421–425.

Raisova, V. (1988). Fiberoptische Laryngoskopie in der phoniatrischen Praxis. *Proceedings of the 15th UEP Congress,* Erlangen, Germany.

Raman, R. S. (1988). Laryngeal examination. *Archives of Otolaryngology-Head and Neck Surgery, 114,* 578–579.

Ramig, L., Scherer, R., & Titze, I. (1989). The aging voice. In V. Lawrence (Ed.), *Transcripts of the 4th Symposium: Care of the Professional Voice* (pp. 131–137). New York: The Voice Foundation.

Ray, C. (1937). *Scientific wonders of the world.* New York: Metro Publications.

Saito, S., Fukuda, H., Kitahara, S., & Kokawa, N. (1978). Stroboscopic observation of vocal fold vibration with fiberoptics. *Folia Phoniatrica, 30,* 241–244.

Schonharl, E. (1960a). *Die Stroboskopie in der praktischen Laryngologie.* Stuttgart: Georg Thieme Verlag.

Sercarz, J. A., Berke, G. S., Arnstein, D., Gerratt, B., & Navidad, M. (1991). A new technique for quantitative measurement of laryngeal videostroboscopic images. *Archives of Otolaryngology and Head and Neck Surgery, 117,* 871–875.

Sercarz, J. A., Berke, G. S., Gerratt, B. R., Kreiman, J., Ming, Y., & Navidad, M. (1992). Synchronizing videostoboscopic images of human laryngeal vibration with physiological signals. *American Journal of Otolaryngology, 13,* 40–44.

Trenque, P. L., & Perrier, P. (1954). *Journal Francaise d'Oto-Rhino-Laryngologie, Audiophonologie et Chirurgie Maxillo-Faciale, 3,* 6.

Vallancien, B. (1954). Le strobophone. *Transactions de la Société de Laryngologie des Hôpitaux de Paris.*

Verhulst, J. L. (1984). La vidéo laryngostropie. *Bordeaux Medical, 17,* 1037–1039.

von Leden, H. V. (1961). The electric synchron-stroboscope: Its value for the practicing laryngologist. *Annals of Otology, Rhinology, and Laryngology, 70,* 881–893.

von Leden, H. V., Moore, P., & Timcke, R. (1960b). Laryngeal vibrations: III. The pathologic larynx. *Archives of Otology, 71,* 1232–1250.

Watanabe, H., Shin, T., & Matsuo, K. (1986). A new computer-analyzing system for clinical use with the strobovideoscope. *Archives of Otolaryngology, 112,* 978–981.

Wendler, J. (1992). Stroboscopy [Special Article]. *Journal of Voice, 6,* 149–154.

Wendler, J., Koppen, K., & Fischer, S. (1987). The validity of stroboscopic data in terms of quantitative measures. *Acta Phoniatrica Latina, 11,* 7–12.

Wendler, J., Koppen, K., Fischer, S., & Cebullar, M. (1988). On the clinical relevance of vibratory parameters in laryngostroboscopy. In *Proceedings of the 15th Union of European Phoniatricians Congress* [Erlangen]. Köln: Deutscher Artze Verlag.

Wendler, J., Otto, C., & Nawka, T. H. (1983). Stroboglottometrie — Eine neues Verfahren zur Schwingungsanalyse der Stimmlippen. *HNO-Praxis, 8,* 263–268.

West, R. (1935). A view of the larynx through a new stroboscope. *Quarterly Journal of Speech, 21,* 355.

Winckel, F. (1954b). Improved stroboscopic technique for examination. *Archiv Ohren-, Nasen-, and Kehlkopf-heilkunde, 165,* 585–586.

Wolfe, R. (1987). *Stroboscopy.* Unpublished manuscript.

Yoshida, Y. (1969). A study of the vibration of the vocal cord with ultra high-speed motion. *Nippon Jibiinkoka Gakkai Kaiko, 72,* 1232–1250.

Yoshida, Y. (1977). An improved model of laryngo-stroboscope. *Otolaryngology, 49,* 663–669.

Yoshida, Y. (1979). A video-tape recording system for laryngostroboscopy. *Journal of the Japan Bronchoesophagological Society, 30*, 1–5.

Yoshida, Y., Hirano, M., & Nakajima, T. (1979). An improved model of laryngo-stroboscope. *Journal of the Japan Bronchoesophagological Society, 30*, 6–12.

Yoshida, Y., Hirano, M., Yoshida, T., & Tateishi, O. (1985). Strobofiberscopic colour video recording of vocal fold vibration. *Journal of Laryngology and Otology, 99*, 795–800.

Zwitman, D. H. (1990). Utilization of transoral endoscopy to assess velopharyngeal closure. *Seminars in Speech and Language, 11*, 38–46.

SURGERY

Cornut, G., & Bouchayer, M. (1971). Apport de la microchirurgie endolaryngée dans le traitement des troubles vocaus. *Journal of Medicine (Lyon)*, 15-25.

Cornut, G., & Bouchayer, M. (1972). Indications phoniatriques de la microchirurgie laryngée. *Journal Français d'Oto Rhino Laryngologie Audiophonologie et Chirurgie Maxillo-Faciale, 22*, 5–52

Cornut, G., & Bouchayer, M. (1973). Apport de la microchirurgie laryngée dans le traitement du nodule de la corde vocale. *Folia Phoniatrica, 24*, 431–437.

Cornut, G., & Bouchayer, M. (1977a). Indications phoniatriques et resultats fonctionnels de la microchirurgie laryngée. *Bulletin d'Audiophonologie, 7*, 5–52.

Cornut, G., & Bouchayer, M. (1977b). Voix et microchirurgie laryngée. *Bulletin d' Audiophonologie, 7*, 5–51.

Cornut, G.,& Bouchayer, M. (1986). Apport de la vidéo stroboscopie dans les indications de phonochirurgie. *Acta Oto-rhino-laryngologica Belgica (Bruxelles), 40*, 436–442.

Cornut, G., Bouchayer, M., & Parent, F. (1986). Value of videostroboscopy in indicating phonosurgery. *Acta Oto-rhino-laryngologica Belgica (Bruxelles), 40*, 436–442.

Cornut, G., Bouchayer, M., & Witzig, E. (1984). Indications phoniatriques et resultats fonctionnels de la microchirurgie laryngée chez l'enfant et l'adolescent. *Bulletin d' Audiophonologie, 17*, 473–496.

Cornut, G., Bouchayer, M., Witzig, E., Roch, J. E., & Laire, R. (1985). Diagnostic et traitement du kyste muqueux par retention de la corde vocale, à propos de 36 cas. *Bulletin d'Audiophonologie, 1*, 263–274.

Fex, S. (1970a). *Experimentel reinnervation av skeletmuskel och den tillämpning vid larynxpareser.* Doctoral dissertation, Technical University of Lund, Sweden.

Hirano, M. (1988). Endolaryngeal microsurgery. In G. M. English (Ed.), *Otolaryngology* (Vol. 3, pp. 1–11). Philadelphia: J. B. Lippincott.

Hirano. M. (1989). Surgical alteration of voice quality. In C. W. Cummings, J. M. Frederickson, L. A. Harker, C. J. Krause, & D. E. Schuller (Eds.), *Otolaryngology Head and Neck Surgery*, (Update 1, pp. 239–264). St. Louis, MO: C. V. Mosby.

Hirano, M., Gould, W. J., Lambiase, A., & Kakita, Y. (1981). Vibratory behavior of the vocal folds in a case with a unilateral polyp. *Folia Phoniatrica, 33*, 275–284.

Kobayashi, S. (1978). Glottal vibration after Hirano's reconstruction following hemilaryngectomy. An ultrahigh speed cinematographic investigation. *Otologia (Fukuoka), 24*, 831–849.

Kume, M. (1975). Microcirurgia estroboscopia de la laringe. *Archivos Medicos del Instituto Mexicano Segura Social, 14*, 20–25.

Maves, M. D., McCabe, B. F., & Gray, S. (1989). Phonosurgery: Indications and pitfalls. *Annals of Otology, Rhinology, and Laryngology, 98*, 577–580.

Milutinovic, Z. (1990). Advantages of indirect videostroboscopic surgery of the larynx. *Folia Phoniatrica, 42*, 77–82.

Saito, S. (1973). Microchirurgie stroboscopique du larynx. *Revue d'Laryngologie, d'Otologie, et de Rhinologie (Bordeaux), 94*, 9–10.

Saito, S. (1977). Phonosurgery. Basic study on the mechanism of phonation and endolaryngeal microsurgery. *Otologia (Fukuoka), 23*, 171–184.

Saito, S., Fukuda, H., & Kitahara, S. (1975). Stroboscopic microsurgery of the larynx. *Archives of Otolaryngology, 101*, 196–201.

Saito, S., Fukuda, H., & Kitahara, S. (1976). Functional microsurgery of the larynx. *Journal of the Japan Bronchoesophagological Society, 27*, 8–16.

Sawashima, M., Totsuka, G., Kobayashi, T., & Hirose, M. (1968). Reconstructive surgery for hoarseness due to unilateral vocal cord paralysis. *Archives of Otolaryngology, 87*, 289.

Schiratzki, H. (1988). Sulcus glottidis. Phonosurgical aspects. *Acta Oto-laryngologica (Stockholm), 449*, 33.

TESTING ISSUES

Baer, T. (1979). Vocal jitter: A neuromuscular explanation. In V. Lawrence (Ed.), *Transcripts of the 8th symposium: Care of the professional voice Part II.* New York: The Voice Foundation.

Baken, J. R. (1987). *Clinical measurement of speech and voice.* Boston: College-Hill Press.

Bastian, R. W. (1987a). Laryngeal image biofeedback for voice disorder patients. *Journal of Voice, 1*, 279–282.

Bastian, R. W. (1987b). Laryngeal videostroboscopy and

photography for the diagnosis and management of voice disorders. *Insights in Otolaryngology, 2.*

Biever, D., & Bless, D. M. (1989). Vibratory characteristics of the vocal folds in young adult and geriatric women. *Journal of Voice, 3,* 120–131.

Biever, D. M., Bless, D. M., & Milenkovic, P. (1990). Acoustic inverse filtering in young and old women. *ASHA, 33,* 63.

Bless, D. M. (1988). Voice disorders in the adult: Assessment. In D. E. Yoder & R. Kent (Eds.), *Decision making in speech-language pathology* (pp. 136–139). Philadelphia: B. C. Decker.

Bless, D. M., & Abbs, J. H. (Eds.). (1983). *Vocal fold physiology.* San Diego, CA: College-Hill Press.

Bless, D. M., & Brandenburg, J. H. (1983, January). *Stroboscopic evaluation of functional voice disorders.* Paper presented at the Middle Section of the Triological Society, Madison, WI.

Bless, D. M., Glaze, L., Lowery, D. B., Campos, G., & Peppard, R. (1990). *Stroboscopic, acoustic and perceptual analysis of voice production in normal speaking adults.* Manuscript in press.

Bless, D. M., Leeper, H. A., & Hirano, M. (1985). *Reliability and validity of stroboscopic judgments.* Unpublished manuscript. University of Wisconsin-Madison, Vocal Function Laboratory.

Booth, J. R., & Childers, D. G. (1979). Automated analysis of ultra high-speed laryngeal films. *IEEE Transactions on Biomedical Engineering, 4,* 185–192.

Bouchayer, M., & Cornut, G. (1974). Kystes et pseudo-kystes de la corde vocale: Propos de 32 cas. *Comptes Rendus des Seances; Congres Français; Societé Française d'Oto-Rhino-Laryngologie et de Pathologie Cervico-Faciale,* 252-259.

Bouchayer, M., & Cornut, G. (1978). Le sulcus glottidis. Notions nouvelles apportees par la microchirurgie laryngée à propos de 31 cas. *Les Cahiers d'Oto Rhino Laryngologie,13,* 769–777.

Bouchayer, M., & Cornut, G. (1984). Les vergetures des cordes vocales. *Revue de Laryngologie, Otologie, Rhinologie (Bordeaux), 105*(4), 421–423.

Bouchayer, M., Cornut, G., Witzig, E., Loire, R., Roch, J. B., & Bastian, R. (1985). Epidermoid cysts, sulci and mucosi bridges of the true vocal cord: A report of 157 cases. *Laryngoscope, 95,* 1087–1094.

Cammann, R. J., Pahn, J., & Rother, U. (1976). Diagnostik der n.-laryngicus-superior-Parese. *Folia Phoniatrica, 28,* 349–353.

Childers, D. G. (1977). Laryngeal pathology detection. *Critical Reviews in Bioengineering, 2,* 375–426.

Childers, D. G., Paige, A., & Moore, P. (1976). Laryngeal vibration patterns. *Archives of Otolaryngology, 102,* 407–410.

Clary (1932). La phonoscope a cordes vibrantes. *Revue Scientifique, 70,* 461.

Colton, R. H. (1972). Phonational range in the modal and falsetto registers. *Journal of Speech and Hearing Research, 15,* 708–713.

Colton, R. H., & Casper, J. K. (1990). *Understanding voice problems: A physiological perspective for diagnosis and treatment.* Baltimore: Williams & Wilkins.

Colton, R. H., Casper, J. K., Brewer, D. W., & Conture, E. G. (1989). Digital processing of laryngeal images: A preliminary report. *Journal of Voice, 3,* 132–142.

Conture, E. G., Schwartz, H., & Brewer, D. W. (1986). Laryngeal behavior during stuttering: A further study. *Journal of Speech and Hearing Research, 28,* 233–240.

Cornut, G., & Bouchayer, M. (1971). Apport de la microchirurgie endolaryngée dans le traitement des troubles vocaus. *Journal of Medicine (Lyon),* 15-25.

Cornut, G.,& Bouchayer, M. (1985). Les therapeutiques phoniatriques de la voix chantée. *Revue de Laryngologie, Otologie, Rhinologie (Bordeaux), 106,* 289–294.

Cornut, G., & Bouchayer, M. (1987). Les troubles de la voix chantée. *O.P.A. Pratique, 11,* 1–4.

Cornut, G., & Bouchayer, M. (1988a). Bilan de quinze années de collaboration entre phoniatre et phono-chirurgien. *Bulletin d'Audiophonologie, 4,* 7–50.

Cornut, G., & Bouchayer, M. (1988b). *Medical instrumentation: video stroboscopy. Assessment of cases for phono-surgery* (p. 6). Stockholm: Brüel et Kjaer.

Cornut, G., & Lafon, J. C. (1960). Vibrations neuromusculaires des cordes vocales et theories de la phonation. *Journal Francais d'Oto Rhino Laryngologie Audiophonologie et Chirurgie Maxillo-Faciale, 9,* 317–324.

Costamagna, D. (1988). *La vidéo-stroboscopie en laryngologie* (Vol. 2, 2nd ed, pp. 132, 230). Nice, France: Thèse Médicine.

Costamagna, D. (1990). La vidéo-laryngostroboscopie. *Bulletin d'Audiophonologie, 6,* 491–546.

Croft, T. A. (1971). Failure of visual estimation of motion under strobe. *Nature, 231,* 397.

Cvejic, D., & Spalajkovic, M. (1964). *Srpski Arkhiv Tselinogradskii Kelkopfheilkunde, 27,* 751.

Damste, H. (1957). Stroboscopic fixation of the vocal cords. *Practica Oto-Rhino-Laryngologica, 19,* 438.

Davis, S. B. (1981). Acoustic characteristics of laryngeal pathology. In J. L. Darby (Ed.), *Speech evaluation in medicine* (pp. 77-104). New York: Grune & Stratton.

Decker, T. N. (1990). *Instrumentation: An introduction for students in the speech and hearing sciences.* New York: Longman.

Dodart, M. (1700). Memoire sur les causes de la Voix de l'Homme, *Histoire de l'Academie des Sciences, 308.*

Dunker, E., & Schlobhauer, B. (1961). Unregelmäsige Stimmlippenschwingungen bei funktionellen Stimmstörungen. *Zeitschrift für Laryngologie und Rhinologie, 40,* 917–934.

Eigler, G., Podzubwit, G., & Weiland, H. (1953). Ein neues mikrophongesteuertes lichtblitz Stroboskop zur Beobachtung von Stimmlippenschwingungen. *Zeitschrift für Laryngologie und Rhinologie, 32,* 40–45.

Eliseyeva, L. P., & Trinos, L. A. (1972). Mobility of true vocal cords in deaf people and in people with low hearing acuity. *Zhurnal Ushnykh Nosovykh Gorlovykh Boleznei, 2,* 25–28.

Emanuel, F., & Sansone, F. (1969). Some spectral features of normal and simulated "rough" vowels. *Folia Phoniatrica, 21,* 401–415.

Ernst, T. (1959). The stroboscopic recognition of functional voice disorders by means of singing and speaking stress. *Archiv für Ohren- Nasen- und Kehlkopfheilkunde, 175,* 452–455.

Ernst, R. (1960). Stroboscopic studies in professional speakers. *HNO, 8,* 170–174.

Faure, M. A., & Muller, A. (1992). Stroboscopy [Special Article]. *Journal of Voice, 6,* 139–148.

Feder, R. J. (1986). On standardizing the laryngeal examination. *Archives of Otolaryngology — Head and Neck Surgery, 112,* 145.

Fenton, E., Niimi, S., Harris, K. S., & Sehley, W. S. (1976, November). *Stroboscopic investigations of larynges of Parkinson's disease patients.* Paper presented at the American Speech and Hearing Association Annual Convention.

Ferrein, A. (1741). De la formation de la voix de l' homme. *Histoire de la Société Royale de Médicine (Paris), 409–432.*

Fex, S. (1970b). Judging the movements of vocal cords in larynx paralysis. *Acta Oto-laryngologica (Stockholm), 263,* 82–83.

Flanagan, J. L., & Ishizaka, K. (1978). Computer model to characterize the air volume displaced by the vibrating vocal cords. *Journal of the Acoustical Society of America, 63,* 1559–1565.

Gall, V. (1984). Strip kymography of the glottis. *Archives of Oto- Rhino- Laryngology, 240,* 287–293.

Gottfried, E. L. (1992). Voice tests and lab tests. Voice and Voice Disorders 3, *American Speech and Hearing Association Newsletter, 2,* 1–3.

Gottfried, E. L., & Wagar, E. A. (1983). Laboratory testing: A practical guide. *Disease-a-Month, 29,* 9.

Gould, W. J. (1984). The clinical voice laboratory. Clini-cal application of voice research. *Annals of Otology, Rhinology, and Laryngology, 93,* 346–350.

Gould, W. J. (1988). The clinical voice laboratory: Clinical application of voice research. *Journal of Voice, 1,* 305–309.

Gould, W. J., & Martin, G. F. (1990). The contribution of the speech sciences to the development of phonosurgery. Personal communication.

Hecker, M., & Kruel, E. (1971). Descriptions of the speech of patients with cancer of the vocal folds. Part 1. Measure of fundamental frequency. *Journal of the Acoustical Society of America, 49,* 1275–1282

Helmholtz, H. (1948). *Sensations of tone* (6th ed., pp. 88–102). New York: Peter Smith.

Hirano, M. (1981a). *Clinical examination of voice.* New York: Springer-Verlag.

Hirano, M., & Hartmann, H. G. (1986). Aspects of videostroboscopy in practice. In *Proceedings of the 20th IALP Congress* (p. 402). Tokyo: The Organizing Committee of the XXth Congress of the International Association of Logopedics and Phoniatrics.

Hirano, M., Hibi, S., Teresawa, R., & Fuciu, M., (1986). Relationship between aerodynamic, vibratory, acoustic, and psychoacoustic correlates in dysphonia. *International Journal of Phonetics, 14,* 445–456.

Hirano, M., Nozoe, I., Shin, T., & Maeyama, T. (1972). Vibration of the vocal cords with recurrent laryngeal nerve palsy. A stroboscopic investigation. *Practica Oto Rhino Laryngologica, 65,* 1037–1047.

Hirano, M., Vennard, W. & Ohala, J. (1970) Regulation of register, pitch, and intensity of voice: An electromyographic investigation of intrinsic laryngeal muscles. *Folia Phoniatrica, 22,* 1–20.

Hirano, M., Yoshida, Y., Matsushita, H., & Nakajima, T. (1974). An apparatus for high speed cinematography of the vocal folds. *Annals of Otology, Rhinology and Laryngology, 83,* 12–18.

Hiroto, I. (1966). The mechanism of phonation, its pathophysiologic aspects. *Oto Rhino Laryngology Clinic, Kyoto, 59,* 229–291.

Hollien, H., & Curtis, J. (1960). A laminographic study of vocal pitch. *Journal of Speech and Hearing Research, 3,* 361.

Holmberg, E., & Leanderson, R. (1983). Laryngeal aerodynamics and voice quality. In V. Lawrence (Ed.), *Transcripts of the Eleventh Symposium on Care of the Professional Voice, Part, II, Medical-Surgical Sessions: Papers.* New York: The Voice Foundation.

Honjo, I., & Isshiki, N. (1980). Laryngoscopic and voice characteristics of aged persons. *Archives of Otolaryngology, 106,* 149–150.

Husson, R. (1951). Stroboscopic study of reflex modifications of vibration of vocal cords produced by experimental stimulations of auditory and trigeminal nerves. *Comptes Rendus de l' Academie Science, Paris,* 232, 1247–1249.

Imaizumi, S. (1986). Spectrographic evaluation of laryngeal pathology. In C.W. Cummings (Ed.), *Otolaryngology-Head and Neck Surgery,* (pp. 1838–1845). St. Louis, MO: C. V. Mosby.

Karnell, M. P. (1989). Synchonized videostroboscopy and electroglottography. *Journal of Voice,* 3, 68–75.

Kitzing, P. (1985). Stroboscopy — A pertinent laryngological examination. *Otolaryngology (London),* 14, 151–175.

Klingholz, F., & Martin, F. (1985). Quantitative spectral evaluation of shimmer and jitter. *Journal of Speech and Hearing Research,* 28, 169–174.

Lehman, J. J., Bless, D. M., & Brandenburg, J. H. (1988). An objective assessment of voice production after radiation therapy for stage I squamous cell carcinoma of the glottis. *Otolaryngology-Head and Neck Surgery,* 98, 121–129.

Liberman, P. (1969). Vocal cord motion in man. *Annals of the New York Academy of Science,* 155, 28–38.

Ludlow, C. (1981). Research needs for the assessment of phonatory function. In C. Ludlow & M. Hart (Eds.), *Proceedings of the Conference on Assessment of Vocal Cord Pathology* (pp. 3–8). Danville, IL: American Speech-Language-Hearing Association.

Maliutin, E. M. (1980). Stroboscopic phenomena in vocal students. *Russkaia Klinika,* 13, 681–691.

Mavlov, L., & Kehaiov, A. (1969). Le rôle des cordes vocales dans la parole scandée et explosive lors de lesions cerebelleuses. *Revue de Laryngologie, d'Otologie, et de Rhinologie (Bordeaux),* 90, 320–324.

Monday, L. A., Bouchayer, M., Cornut, G., & Roch, J. B. (1983). Epidermoid cysts of the vocal cords. *Annals of Otology, Rhinology, and Laryngology,* 92, 124–127.

Monday, L. A., Cornut, G., Bouchayer, M., Roch, J. B., & Loire, R. (1981). Diagnosis and treatment of intracordal cysts. *Journal of Otolaryngology (Toronto),* 10, 363–370.

Moore, D. M., Berle, S., Hanson, D. G., & Ward, P. H. (1987). Videostroboscopy of the canine larynx. The effects of asymmetric laryngeal tension. *Laryngoscope,* 97, 543–553.

Moore, D. M., & von Leden, H. (1958). Dynamic variations of the vibratory pattern in the normal larnyx. *Folia Phoniatrica,* 10, 205–238.

Musehold, A. (1898). Stroboskopische und photographische Studien über die Stellung der Stimmlippen im Brust und Falsett-register. *Archiv für Laryngology und Rhinology,* 7, 1–21.

National Institute for Deafness and Other Communication Disorders. (1990, September). *Assessment of speech and voice production: Research and clinical applications.* Monograph, Proceedings of a Conference, Bethesda, MD.

Ohyama, M., Ohno, I., Fujita, T., & Adachi, K. (1981). Surface ultrastructures of the human laryngeal mucosa. Observation by a newly developed technique of SEM cinematography. *Biomedical Research,* 2, 273–279.

Pascher, W., & Johannsen, H. S. (1975). Angewandte phoniatrie. I. Methodik der Stimmuntersuchung. *HNO,* 23, 84–90.

Pederson, M. F., & Boberg, A. (1973). Examination of voice function of patients with paralysis of the recurrent nerve. *Acta Oto-laryngologica (Stockholm),* 75, 372–374.

Peppard, R. C., & Bless, D. M. (1990). A method for improving measurement reliability in laryngeal videostroboscopy. *Journal of Voice,* 4, 280–285.

Peppard, R., Bless, D. M., & Milenkovic, P. (1988). Comparison of young adult singers and nonsingers with vocal nodules. *Journal of Voice,* 2, 250–260.

Perello, J. (1962). La théorie muco-ondulatoire de la phonation. *Annales d'Oto-laryngologie et Chirurgie Cervico-Faciale,* 79, 722–725.

Rakhmilevich, A. G., & Lavrova, E. V. (1971). Phonopedic therapy and stroboscopy of patients with affection of the inferior laryngeal nerve. *Otorhinolaryngology,* 33, 10–12.

Rammage, L. A., Peppard, R. C., & Bless, D. M. (1992). Aerodynamic, laryngoscopic, and perceptual-acoustic characteristics in dysphonic females with posterior glottal chinks: A retrospective study. *Journal of Voice,* 6, 64–78.

Remacle, M., Marbaix, E., & Bertrand, B. (1986). Emploi du collagène injectable pour la réhabilitation vocale et glottique. *Les Cahiers d'Oto Rhino Laryngologie,* 21, 169–178.

Remacle, M., & Millet, B. (1987). Recurrent nerve paralysis after thyroidectomy. Therapeutic approach. *Acta Oto Rhino Laryngologica Belgica (Bruxelles),* 41, 910–916.

Remorino, A. (1955). *Annales de Fonologie et d'Audiologie,* 1, 100.

Roche, J. B., Bouchayer, M., & Cornut, G. (1981). Le sulcus glottidis. *Revue de Laryngologie, d'Otologie, et de Rhinologie (Bordeaux),* 102, 333–346.

Rontal, E., Rontal, H., & Rolnick, M. I. (1983). Objective evaluation of vocal pathology using voice spectrography. *Annales d'Otolaryngologie et de Chirurgie Cervico-Faciale, 84*, 662–671.

Rossi, M., Raso, D. Y., & Disceglie, P. (1968). *Clinica Oto Rhino Laryngologica, 20*, 740.

Rothenberg, M. (1973). A new inverse-filtering technique for deriving the glottal airflow during waveform during voicing. *Journal of the Acoustical Society of America, 53*, 1632–1645.

Russell, G. O., & Tuttle, C. H. (1930). Color movies of vocal cord action aid in diagnosis. *Laryngoscope, 40*, 549–552.

Sataloff, R. T. (1987b). The professional voice: Part I. Anatomy, function, and general health. *Journal of Voice, 1*, 92–104.

Sataloff, R. T. (1987c). The professional voice: Part II. Physical examination. *Journal of Voice, 1*, 191–201.

Sataloff, R. T., Spiegel, J. R., Carroll, L. M., Darby, K. S., Hawkshaw, M. J., & Rulnick, R. K. (1990). The clinical voice laboratory: Practical design and practical application. *Journal of Voice, 4*, 264–279.

Schearer, W. M. (1984). Academic and instructional applications for microcomputers. In A. H. Schwartz (Ed.), *The handbook of microcomputer applications in communication disorders* (pp. 193–219). San Diego: College-Hill Press.

Scherer, R. C., Gould, W. J., Titze, I. R., Meyers, A. D., & Sataloff, R. T. (1988). Preliminary evaluation of selected acoustic and glottographic measures for clinical phonatory function analysis. *Journal of Voice, 2*, 230–244.

Schiratzki, H. (1988). Sulcus glottidis. Phonosurgical aspects. *Acta Oto-laryngologica (Stockholm), 449*, 33.

Schonharl, E. (1954). Stroboscopic study in myxedema. *Archivs für Ohren-, Nasen-, und Kehlkopfheilkunde, 165*, 633–635.

Schonharl, E. (1960a). *Die Stroboskopie in der praktischen Laryngologie.* Stuttgart: Georg Thieme Verlag.

Schuerenberg, B., & Moser, M. (1986). Entwicklung und derzeitiger Stand der TV-farb-stroboskopie. *Proceedings of the 13th UEP Congress* (p. 24), Vienna.

Schutte, H., & Seidner, W. (1983). Recommendation by the Union of European Phoniatricians (UEP): Standardizing voice measurement/phonetography. *Folia Phoniatrica, 35*, 286–288.

Segre, R. (1933). Vocal nodules as revealed by stroboscope. *Valsalva, 9*, 380–389.

Sercarz, J. A., Berke, G. S., Arnstein, D., Gerratt, B., & Navidad, M. (1991). A new technique for quantitative measurement of laryngeal videostroboscopic images. *Archives of Otolaryngology and Head and Neck Surgery, 117*, 871–875.

Sercarz, J. A., Berke, G. S., Gerratt, B. R., Kreiman, J.,

Ming, Y., & Navidad, M. (1992a). Synchronizing videostroboscopic images of human laryngeal vibration with physiological signals. *American Journal of Otolaryngology, 13*, 40–44.

Shin, Y. (1976). Clinical and pathological investigations of sulcus vocalis. *Otologia (Fukuoka), 22*, 819–835.

Shipp, T. (1973). Intra-oral airpressure and lip occlusion in midvocalic stop consonant production. *Journal of Phonetics, 1*, 167–170.

Shipp, T. (1987). Vertical laryngeal position: Research findings and application for singers. *Journal of Voice, 1*, 217–221.

Shipp, T. Guinn, L., Sundberg, J., & Titze, I. T. (1987). Vertical laryngeal positioning: Research findings and their relationship to singing. *Journal of Voice, 1*, 220–222.

Shipp, T., & McGlone, R. (1971). Laryngeal dynamics associated with voice frequency change. *Journal of Speech and Hearing Research, 14*, 761–768.

Simpson, I. C. (1971). Dysphonia: The organization and working of a dysphonia clinic. *British Journal of Disorders of Communication, 6*, 70–85.

Smith, S. (1954). Remarks on the physiology of the vibrations of the vocal cords. *Folia Phoniatrica, 6*, 166–178.

Smith, S. (1957). Chest register versus head register in the membrane cushion model of the vocal cords. *Folia Phoniatrica, 9*, 32–36.

Smith, S. (1959). Le jet d'air relatif aux mouvements des cordes vocales des deux modeles. *Journal Français d'Oto-Rhino-Laryngologie, d'Audiophonologie et de Chirurgie Maxillo-Faciale, 8*, 113–118.

Smitheran, J., & Hixon, T. (1971). A clinical method for estimating laryngeal airway resistance during vowel production. *Journal of Speech and Hearing Disorders, 46*, 138–146.

Sonneburg, A., Giger, M., Kern, L., Noll, C., Stuby, K., Weber, K. B., & Blum, A. L. (1979). How reliable is determination of ulcer size by endoscopy? *British Medical Journal, 280*, 1322.

Sonninen, A. (1970). Phoniatric viewpoints on hoarseness. *Acta Oto-laryngologica (Stockholm), 263*, 68–81.

Stelzig, G. (1988). Schwingungsmuster bei neurologischen Grunderkrankungen. *Proceedings of the 15th Union of European Phoniatricians* [Erlangen]. Köln: Deutsche Artze Verlag.

Stern, H. (1931). Eine kurze Zusammenfassung des derzeitigen Standes der Frage der Beruteuilung und Bewertung stroboskopischer Befunde für die Pathologie der Stimme. *Monatsschrift für Ohrenheilkunde und Laryngo-Rhinologie, 65*, 691–702.

Stevens, K. N. (1977). Physics of laryngeal behavior and larynx modes. *Phonetica, 34*, 264–279.

Stoicheff, M. (1981). Speaking fundamental frequency characteristics of nonsmoking female adults. *Journal of Speech and Hearing Research, 24,* 437–441.

Tanabe, M., Kitajima, K., Gould, W. J., & Lambiase, A. Analysis of high-speed motion pictures of the vocal folds. *Folia Phoniatrica, 27,* 77–87.

Tarneaud, J. L. (1932). Les dyskinésies de la parole and du chant. *Annals d'Otolaryngologie et de Chirurgie Cervico-Faciale,* 864–890.

Teitler, N. (1992). *Examiner bias: Influence of patient history on perceptual ratings of videostroboscopy.* Unpublished master's thesis, University of Wisconsin-Madison.

Thumfart, F. (1988). From larynx to vocal ability. New electrophysiological data. *Acta Oto-laryngologica (Stockholm), 105,* 425–431.

Timcke, R., von Leden, H., & Moore, P. (1959). Laryngeal vibrations: II. Physiologic vibrations. *Archives of Otolaryngology, 69,* 438–444.

Titze, I. (1981). Biomechanics and distributed-mass models of vocal fold vibration. In K. N. Stevens & M. Hirano (Eds.), *Vocal fold physiology* (pp. 245–250). Tokyo: University of Tokyo Press.

Titze, I. (1988). The physics of small-amplitude oscillation of the vocal folds. *Journal of the Acoustical Society of America, 83,* 1536–1552.

Titze, I. (1989). Physiologic and acoustic differences between male and female voices. *Journal of the Acoustical Society of America, 85,* 1699–1707.

Titze, I. (1990). Interpretation of the electroglottographic signal. *Journal of Voice, 4,* 1–9.

Titze, I., & Scherer, R. (Eds.). (1984). *Biomechanics and acoustics of vocal fold vibration.* Denver: Denver Performing Arts Center.

Titze, I., & Strong, W. J. (1975). Normal modes in vocal cord tissues. *Journal of the Acoustical Society of America, 57,* 736–744.

Titze, I., & Sundberg, J. (1990). *Acoustic power in speech and singing.* Manuscript submitted for publication.

van den Berg, J. W. (1953). *Physica van de stemvorming.* Thèse, University of Gröningen.

van den Berg, J. W. (1958). Myoelastic aerodynamic theory of voice production. *Journal of Speech and Hearing Research, 1,* 227–244.

van den Berg, J. W. (1959). Results of experiments with human larynges. *Practica Oto-Rhino-Laryngologica, 21,* 355.

van den Berg, J. W., Zantema, J. T., & Doornenbal, J. R. (1957). On the air resistance and the Bernouilli effect for the human larynx. *Journal of the Acoustical Society of America, 29,* 626–631.

Vallancien, B. (1955). Effects of various drugs on the action potential of the vestibular nerve in the frog. *Journal Français d'Oto-Rhino-Laryngologie Audiophonologie et Chirurgie Maxillo-Faciale, 17,* 157–163.

Vallancien, B. (1958). Le larynx et sa fonction phonatoire. *Journal Français d'Oto-Rhino-Laryngologie Audiophonologie et Chirurgie Maxillo-Faciale, 7,* 135.

Vallencian, B. (1968). Radiologic study of phonation: The clinical aspect. *Folia Phoniatrica, 20,* 156–181.

Vallancien, B. (1971). Comparison des signaux microphoniques, diaphanographiques et glottographiques avec application au laryngographe. *Folia Phoniatrica, 23,* 371–380.

Vallancien, B. (1972). Progres en exploration fonctionnelle de larynx. *Journal Français d-Oto-Rhino-Laryngologie Audiophonologie et Chirurgie Maxillo-Faciale, 21,* 649–662.

Vasilenko, Y. S. (1972). Significance of individucal indices of vibratory cycle of the vocal folds in general assessment of the stroboscopic picture. *Vestnik Oto-rino-laryngologii (Moskva), 34,* 63–68.

von Leden, H. V. (1961). The electric synchron-stroboscope: Its value for the practicing laryngologist. *Annals of Otology, Rhinology, and Laryngology, 70,* 881–893.

von Leden, H. V. (1971). Übersichten neuere Funktionsteste der Larynx. *HNO, 19,* 225–231.

von Leden, H. V. (1988) Microlaryngoscopy: A historical vignette. *Journal of Voice, 1,* 341–346.

von Leden, H. V., Moore, P., & Timcke, R. (1960a). Laryngeal vibrations: Measurements of the glottic wave. *Archives of Otolaryngology, 71,* 16–35.

von Leden, H. V., Moore, P., & Timcke, R. (1960b). Laryngeal vibrations: III. The pathologic larynx. *Archives of Otology, 71,* 1232–1250.

Weismer, G. (1984). Acoustic analysis of dysarthric speech: Perceptual correlates and physiological inferences. In J. C. Rosenbeck (Ed.), *Seminars in Speech, Hearing and Language, 5,* 293–314.

Wendler, J. (1988). Consideraciones sobre una instrumentacion razonnable para el diagnostico de voz en la practica clinica. *Revue Logopaedia Foniatrica et Audiologica, 8,* 49–53.

Wendler, J., Otto, C., & Nawka, T. H. (1983). Stroboglottometrie — Eine neues Verfahren zur Schwingungsanalyse der Stimmlippen. *HNO-Praxis, 8,* 263–268.

Wendler, J., & Seidner, W. (1987). *Lehrbuch der phoniatrie* (2nd Aufl.). Leipzig, VEB Thieme.

Wendler, J., & Seidner, W. (1988). Methoden und Ergebnisse der Phonochirurgie. *Zeitschrift für Klinische Medizin, 46,* 101–103.

Wendler, J., Seidner, W., & Rose, A. (1973). Zur praktischen Nomenklatur der funktionellen Dysphonien. *Folia Phoniatrica, 25,* 30–38.

Wendler, J., & Vollprecht, I. (1984). Stimmlippen Praxis. *Folia Phoniatrica, 36,* 74–83.

Wilson, F., & Star, C. (1985). Use of the phonation analyzer as a clinical tool. *Journal of Speech and Hearing Disorders, 50,* 351–356.

Winckel, F. (1954a). Neuentwicklung eines Lichtblitz-Stroboskops für die laryngologie. *HNO, 4,* 210.

Winckel, F. (1957). Hörmässige Bewertung von lautanalytischen Ergebnissen. *Zeitschrift für Laryngologie, Rhinologie, Otologie, und ihre Grenzgebiete, 36,* 564–569.

Wolfe, V., & Steinfatt, T. (1987). Prediction of vocal severity within and across voice types. *Journal of Speech and Hearing Research, 30,* 230–240.

Woo, P., Colton, R., Casper, J., & Brewer, D. (1990). Dysphonia in the aging: Physiology vs. disease. *Laryngoscope, 102,* 139–144.

Woo, P., Colton, R., & Shangold, L. (1987). Phonatory airflow analysis in patients with laryngeal disease. *Annals of Otology, Rhinology, and Laryngology, 96,* 549–555.

Yamoto, E., Sasaki, Y., & Okamura, H. (1984). Harmonics-to-noise ratio and psychophysical measurement of the degree of hoarseness. *Journal of Speech and Hearing Research, 27,* 2–6.

Yanagihara, N. (1967). Significance of harmonic changes and noise components in hoarseness. *Journal of Speech and Hearing Research, 10,* 531–541.

Yanagisawa, E. (1983). Videolaryngoscopy: A comparison of fiberscopic and telescopic documentation. *Annals of Otology, Rhinology, and Laryngology, 92,* 430–436.

Yanagisawa, E. (1984). Videolaryngoscopy using a low cost home video system color camera. *Journal of Biological Photography, 52,* 430.

Yanagisawa, E., Casuccio, J. R., & Suzuki, M. (1981). Videolaryngoscopy using a rigid telescope and video home system color camera. *Annals of Otology, Rhinology, and Laryngology, 90,* 346–350.

Yanagisawa, E., Godley, F., & Muta, H. (1987). Selection of video cameras for stroboscopic videolaryngoscopy. *Annals of Otology, Rhinology, and Laryngology, 96,* 578–585.

Yanagisawa, E., Owens, T. W., Strothers, G., & Honda, K. (1983). Videolaryngoscopy: A comparison of fiberscopic and telescopic documentation. *Annals of Otology, Rhinology, and Laryngology, 92,* 430–436.

Yoshida, Y. (1979). A video-tape recording system for laryngostroboscopy. *Journal of the Japan Bronchoesophagological Society, 30,* 1–5.

Yumoto, E., Gould, W. J., & Baer, T. (1982). Harmonics-to-noise ratio as an index of the degree of hoarseness. *Journal of the Acoustical Society of America, 71,* 1544–1550.

Zemlin, R. W. (1988). *Speech and hearing science: Anatomy and physiology* (3rd ed.). Englewood Cliffs, NJ: Prentice-Hall.

Index